Feeling Fabulous

About the Author

Ruth Langsford is one of the UK's most recognised and loved television presenters, with a career spanning over thirty years. A long-time fashion lover, she's built a successful clothing brand on QVC and is a champion of mid-life confidence in women, promoting positivity and self-belief through her Feeling Fabulous brand.

Feeling Fabulous

Be your best self, no matter
what life throws at you

Ruth Langsford

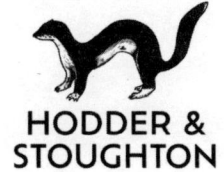

**HODDER &
STOUGHTON**

First published in Great Britain in 2026 by Hodder & Stoughton Limited
An Hachette UK company

The authorised representative in the EEA is Hachette Ireland, 8 Castlecourt Centre, Dublin 15, D15 XTP3, Ireland (email: info@hbgi.ie)

1

Copyright © Ruth Langsford 2026

The right of Ruth Langsford to be identified as the Author of the Work has been asserted by her in accordance with the Copyright, Designs and Patents Act 1988.

All rights reserved. No part of this publication may be reproduced, stored in a retrieval system, or transmitted, in any form or by any means without the prior written permission of the publisher, nor be otherwise circulated in any form of binding or cover other than that in which it is published and without a similar condition being imposed on the subsequent purchaser.

A CIP catalogue record for this title is available from the British Library

Hardback ISBN 9781399756990
ebook ISBN 9781399757027

Typeset in Electra by Hewer Text UK Ltd, Edinburgh
Printed and bound in Great Britain by Clays Ltd, Elcograf S.p.A.

Hodder & Stoughton policy is to use papers that are natural, renewable and recyclable products and made from wood grown in sustainable forests. The logging and manufacturing processes are expected to conform to the environmental regulations of the country of origin.

Hodder & Stoughton Limited
Carmelite House
50 Victoria Embankment
London EC4Y 0DZ

www.hodder.co.uk

For my darling parents, Dennis & Joan

Contents

Prologue: Feeling Fabulous   ix

1   Home Is Where the Heart Is   1
2   Good Girls Don't Get Expelled   11
3   What's the Worst That Can Happen?   25
4   Imposter Syndrome   37
5   Maybe Baby   45
6   Being a Working Mum (the juggle of guilt)   55
7   What's the Worst That Can Happen in Sequins?   65
8   Thanks for the Memories   83
9   When Endings Become Beginnings (in three parts)   105
10   She Looks Good . . . For Her Age   121
11   At My Time of Life   137
12   Sister, Dear Sister   145
13   Loose Women, Lovely Friends   157
14   Fashionista   169
15   When Your Confidence Goes AWOL   181
16   On Being Fabulous   195

Acknowledgements   205

Prologue: Feeling Fabulous

Well, hello you!

What a treat it is to welcome you to *Feeling Fabulous*, something I have been wanting to write for quite some time, and which may just turn out to be your new favourite read. Or, if that's too forward, at least a good book to keep on your bedside table and return to as and when you need it. While it's a pleasure and a privilege to bring my life into yours through these pages rather than the TV screen, it's also a little nerve-racking to be as open and candid as I have been here. But I think the time is right.

So, first things first – can we just take a moment to say it out loud? We made it. Into the murky depths of middle age (and when does that start and end, I wonder?). Past the noise of youth. Past the pressure to pretend we've got it all figured out. Past the expectation to be someone that we are not. And you know what? I reckon this is just the beginning, because I believe with all my heart (and quite a bit of lived experience) that this isn't the winding-down bit. Now is the time to ramp it up. Are you with me?!

Before we go any further, let me make something very clear: I am not an expert in how to feel fabulous. I haven't got a glittering diploma in confidence, and I don't float around with a Pilates mat all day. I'm just Ruth – from the telly, yes, but also from the supermarket queue, the pile of admin and the back of the wardrobe where I've been known to have a little cry over a pair of jeans that no longer fit. I'm just Ruth who pops a curler in her fringe whenever she is cooking and then forgets to take it out before she goes on a dog walk. *That* Ruth.

Just like you, I've lived a life, and it turns out we don't win any medals or get a prize for doing so! But we do have a mental filing cabinet full of all the messy bits, marvellous parts, and everything in between. And this book? It's a celebration of all that – the wins, the wobbles, and the wisdom I have gathered along the way. In telling my story, it may resonate and even help someone else in similar situations. That's my hope, at least!

If I have any qualification to write this book, beyond my experiences so far, it is that I am a glass-half-full kind of girl. I always have been, just like my dear dad. No matter what life has thrown at me over the years (much of it shared in the forthcoming chapters), I pick myself up, brush myself down and start all over again. I believe in the power of positivity and how important it is for all of us to look at things through optimistic rose-tinted glasses. Like the sort that Elton John would be proud to wear: maybe heart-shaped, studded with rhinestones and caked in glitter. Let's put these on and see how much brighter and happier the world looks.

I don't want to sound too frivolous because as well as cramming in the joy, luck and attitude of gratitude, this book takes some sharp turns and traumatic dives, just like my life. It doesn't

Prologue: Feeling Fabulous

always make for easy reading, but as we know well by now, there is still light to be found among the shade.

'Feeling fabulous' started as a fun little phrase I used, which has taken on a much deeper meaning for me in the last couple of years. It's a mantra, a pep talk and an affirmation in one sparkly flourish. More than occasionally, it seems, we need reminding of all that hard-won wisdom to give us more confidence in ourselves. So . . .

- If you've ever looked in the mirror and wondered where you have gone, this book is for you.
- If you've ever carried the weight of failure and imposter syndrome, then this book is for you.
- If you've ever wondered 'what if?', this book might be for you.
- If you've ever felt the tug between your parents, your children, your career, your partner and your own space, I think this book is for you.
- If you've ever experienced searing, life-altering loss, this book could be for you.
- If you've ever stood in your knickers, holding a top in one hand and your will to live in the other, wondering what the hell to wear – oh this book is definitely for you.

You see, something wonderful happens when you stop chasing who you think you should be and start loving who you are right now. That's where the magic lives. Not in wrinkle creams or crash diets or pretending you have boundless energy 24/7. No – it lives in being honest, kind to yourself, and maybe a little bit bold. Because there's no rule book for feeling fabulous, but if there was, it certainly wouldn't say 'must look twenty-five forever'. It would say things like . . .

- Speak up.
- Listen to your gut.
- Eat the cake.
- Don't save the expensive lipstick for best.
- Be as kind to yourself as you are to others.
- Know when to stay and when to quit.
- Say 'no' without apology and 'yes' without guilt.
- Surround yourself with people who lift your spirit rather than crush it.

Feeling fabulous doesn't just cover the physical aspects of my life, it's the emotional ones too, the stuff that digs deeper than a good haircut and a fresh manicure. It goes beyond a nice pair of boots and a stylish handbag. Yes, it includes all those material things (which is great, because I'm a big fan of them), but it also considers the more intangible elements that make me feel good. Like having a sense of purpose, spending time with family and friends, practising gratitude every day and accepting myself for who the hell I am! And if they work for me, then they might make you feel the same way. We may have different desires and dreams, but we are all after the same goal of happiness and contentment. And a bloody good pair of jeans.

One of the reasons I wrote *Feeling Fabulous* was that in all my chats with women over the years – in TV studios, at events,

Prologue: Feeling Fabulous

during a food shop, on social media, and with my friends – one thing kept coming up: so many of us spend our mid-life playing small. Putting others first. Saying 'I'm fine' when we're anything but, and I just thought, enough is enough. It's our time. Not in a selfish, throw-our-toys-out-of-the-pram kind of way, but in a joyful, fantastic, arms-spread-wide way.

I don't just want to be OK, or fine, or to bob along in life. I want the full adventure, which I know means embracing change and the lows as well as the highs, because the lows I have experienced have also shown me where hope lies. Like battling through a rainstorm and then following a rainbow to a pot of gold. Feeling fabulous is as much a state of mind as a practical achievement – in fact, it is mostly about how we view ourselves. It's not just about finding the perfect lipstick (although that is a quest of mine), it encapsulates strength, courage, confidence, humour, resilience, faith and acceptance.

I realise that this is easier said than done, particularly in the face of the most difficult times like divorce, illness and loss, but I have learned a lot as I've navigated those terrible periods. It may sound like a cliché, but a positive mental attitude goes an awfully long way – it's been a sanity saver for me. So too does knowing that I am not alone and that there are countless others who have been through the worst and come out the other side, into the warmth of the sun.

By recounting key stories in my life, from childhood all the way through to my mid-sixties, I can share some of the lessons I have learned. I look at my nomadic childhood, my rebellious teenage years, the way I fell into a job that became my career, my approach to motherhood and the empty nest, the end of things like relationships and finding a new, surprising string to my bow later in life. Here is the last sixty-plus years of what work, love, family, home, friendship and heartbreak mean to me.

As well as my musings and memories, I want you to think of this book as a fabulous toolkit, where we get stuck into some of the thoughts that keep us awake at night. In revealing my perspective on confidence, imposter syndrome and how to stop giving a monkey's about what other people think, I hope it will give you tips on how to do the same. I'll share some of my own 'oops' moments, from body image anxiety to everyday dithering, because believe me, even after all these years, I still get nervous, still overthink, still have those 'is it just me?' days. But I've also learned how to pick myself up again and, after all, what's the worst that can happen?!

We'll also have some fun with fashion and beauty. This isn't about trying to turn back time. It's about style that makes you feel powerful, playful, and utterly you. I want to highlight the joy of a great outfit. There'll be no 'age-appropriate' nonsense or forced body confidence here, just some inspiration to help you celebrate who you are. Because style isn't about dressing young – it's about dressing you. Same goes for beauty – it's not about erasing lines, it's about embracing the face that's loved, laughed, and lived . . . and possibly had one too many Proseccos the night before.

This book is also about BEING fabulous and stepping (running, jumping, skipping) into the joy of living – through trying new things, wearing what we want, dipping into exercise, eating

Prologue: Feeling Fabulous

well, loosening our waistbands and not waiting for permission. Along the way, I'll also talk about the brilliant women I am surrounded by, like my friends, my telly colleagues and my mum, Joan, who always has something wise (and hilarious) to say.

This is where we get our sparkle back, not because we're trying to impress anyone, but because it just feels good. Ultimately, feeling fabulous isn't about becoming someone new – it's about returning to ourselves. The you that got a bit buried under life's to-do lists, expectations, and bras that dig in. I want you to come away from these pages feeling seen, heard, and ready to shine.

So, stick the kettle on. Grab a packet of biscuits or cake (a chocolate eclair for me, please) and let's get ready for a good dose of laughter, thought-provoking chat and maybe the odd tear. We're in this together – and together, we're fabulous. Now go on, turn the page . . . I can't wait to start this journey with you.

With love, gratitude and fabulousness,

Ruth x

1
Home Is Where the Heart Is

When I'm asked where I'm from, I don't really know how to answer. It's easier to say London because that's where I went to school from the age of seven and it's the place I've had the most consistent relationship with throughout my life, but the truth is I don't feel like I come from any one place in particular. My dad was in the army, so we moved around a lot as a family. My sister, Julia, was born in Germany and then I arrived a couple of years later when they were stationed in Southeast Asia before we returned to the UK when I was six months old. From Singapore to Scunthorpe! That could have been a good alternative title for this book.

Wherever we laid our hats, Mum skilfully turned it into a home. The army had a rule about the size and number of wooden crates we were allowed to move around with, so we were quite restricted about what we could take, and this made Mum an expert at organisation and packing. Our belongings were squeezed tightly into boxes emblazoned with 'Langsford' and shipped off to the next base, ready to be unpacked into the regulation-style quarters with its standard army-issue furniture. Every flat and house looked pretty much the same, a blank canvas until my mum arrived with her collection of blankets and cushions to throw over the sofa and chairs. She was a magpie, collecting little treasures from each country we lived in, which told a story of our travels, and she still has some of them now.

I thought this was how everyone lived, moving on to pastures new every two years. I didn't know any different and I certainly didn't stop to analyse our lifestyle as I was busy being a happy, well-adjusted kid. Each house was a home to me because my parents and my sister were there, and we were surrounded by our own things. I felt loved and safe no matter where we were.

Many years later the four of us were reminiscing about the army days, telling stories around the dinner table of countries and houses we had briefly settled in. It was fascinating to hear my parents share their adult perspective on things while my sister and I wore the rose-tinted glasses of childhood nostalgia.

'Oh my God, Dennis, do you remember those awful quarters in Oxford?' Mum said, throwing her hands up in horror. 'We turned up with all our belongings, and the house was absolutely filthy!'

'Yes! Terrible! It stank of dog wee. Do you remember that, girls?' Dad looked from me to my sister, surprised by our confused faces.

'No, where was that?' We didn't remember there ever being a problem anywhere we moved to.

'You know, the one in Oxford!' our parents chorused and shook their heads in disgust at the memory of it.

Home Is Where the Heart Is

And do you know, I do remember arriving at the Oxford house, but it's a very different memory from the one my parents had. It was winter and already dark, and Julia and I were put straight into the bath. Mum had pegged our pyjamas in front of an electric fire, so they were toasty warm when we climbed into them, and we drank mugs of Horlicks before being tucked into bed. We drifted off to sleep while, unbeknown to us, our parents had begun the deep clean, staying up for much of the night to bleach everything they could get their hands on. The realisation that our parents had protected us from that, and that we had no idea until many years later, was another example of an untroubled childhood.

I loved army life. I liked all the moving around, the different places, the foreignness of things in other countries. My earliest memories were of living in Scunthorpe, where we settled when we came back from Singapore. Julia was at school but I wasn't old enough, so Mum and I would take her every morning and then we would go back to piek her up at the end of the day. While she had her head stuck in boring times tables, I was at home surrounded by her toys, knowing she wasn't there to tell me off if I played with something I shouldn't. One time I took a turn on her bike, which I was absolutely not allowed to do, and I fell off into a patch of stinging nettles. What do they say about karma being a bitch?!

Dad was working nearby and came home for lunch every day, so I would wait, watching out of the window for him to walk up the garden path. It was from there that we moved to the filthy, stinky house in Oxford and then it was my turn to start school just before we headed off again.

Dad's next posting was to Tripoli in Libya when I was five. He went ahead of us, which he often did, and when we arrived at the new flat he had left a teddy on each of our beds, along with snorkels and flippers. I was thrilled, even though I had no idea what they were. I'd never seen this sort of kit before and couldn't wait to try it out. I just had to learn to swim first, which was a minor detail.

My teacher at my new school was young, blonde and very pretty, with a stack of silver bangles up each arm that tinkled when she played the piano every morning. The school day was rather different from the one in the UK, partly because it was so hot. Lessons would be in the cool of early morning, then at lunchtime the mums would pick us up and take us straight to the beach. The dads would finish work in the afternoon and come down to join us. I couldn't imagine a better way to live!

Our family embraced the lifestyle, and we spent a lot of time on the beach, as proved by all the photographs – so many photographs! – from that time showing Dad soaking up the sun, his Cornish genes turning him as brown as a berry. And red-headed, fair-skinned Mum in the background, wearing a hat, a towel covering her legs, sitting under a large umbrella while we ran about without a care in the world. We didn't know about the dangers of too much sun in those days and would have the barest smear of sun cream. I now go twice a year to have my moles checked.

I have vivid flashes of memory from this time. My first taste of a weird and wonderful fruit called watermelon. Seeing bananas growing on trees near our flat. The intensity of the heat. The dust (oh my goodness the dust) in the air, on our clothes and coating the car. Dad had bought a big second-hand American station wagon with one long bench seat in the front, which was quite an eccentric choice, but I thought it was so cool. He also treated himself to his dream Rolex Submariner watch, as it was duty-free and much cheaper. I was fascinated by it because he would dive into the water still wearing it. He taught us to swim while we were in Tripoli, so our snorkels and flippers got a lot of use.

What our photo albums from that time don't show is the undercurrent of tension that was building. The Libyans wanted the British army out. While we children were mostly oblivious, our parents were very aware of the growing unrest. One day, we were standing at the bus stop outside our block of flats, me holding one of Mum's hands and Julia holding the other, and a man cycled past and hissed at us. Mum gently pulled us back from the road, tucking us behind her. I think I remember this, but it could be one of those events that I had been told about and so it etched itself second hand into my memory bank.

We left Tripoli slightly sooner than we were supposed to as the political climate shifted and we moved straight to Berlin, swapping intense heat for freezing cold. There was thick snow on the ground when we arrived, and I was captivated by it.

My parents, then in their thirties, had the most fantastic time there. It was the mid-sixties, and they became the best of friends with their neighbours, Arthur and Rosa, who we called (and still call) Uncle and Auntie. Their social life was full of trips to restaurants, the theatre and the opera, made easier by the fact that they were child free for long periods of time because Julia and I, aged ten and seven, were off at boarding school, back in England.

Our family lived in three different places in Germany – Berlin, Celle, an historic town of half-timbered houses set on the banks of the river Aller, and Bielefeld, one of the largest cities in the country – before Dad was posted to Malta. I loved it because it was hot, and we had an amazing apartment overlooking Sliema Bay and the old town. I had my first boy crush there: he was the blond brother of a friend of mine who was paid to take us to the cinema, but I decided we were on a date even though he didn't speak to me and sat four seats away. Another time, I arrived home for the school holidays with a head full of nits and spent hours sitting on the balcony while Mum combed the ghastly shampoo through my hair. Julia was so fascinated she got a live one and put it under the microscope from her science kit to have a closer look.

Weekends as a boarder were fun and filled with the same sort of stuff we would have done if we were at home, like reading magazines, shopping and listening to records. Those weekends when we were allowed to go home were trickier for Julia and me because it was too far and costly. We would occasionally go and stay with Uncle Arthur and Auntie Rosa, who had moved back to the UK by then. Julia was in charge of our safe travel from London, which was a responsibility that weighed heavily on her and one she wasn't really old enough for. Once, as we pulled into the train station Uncle Arthur was collecting us from, we found we were in the wrong carriage as the platform was too short. Committed to getting us to our destination, Julia flung open the door, chucked our suitcases out and told me to jump as if we were parachuting from a plane. Uncle Arthur was perturbed to see us rolling in the dusty sidings.

For half-term holidays, we stayed with our grandmother in her cosy council flat in Portsmouth. I loved my grandma and Patch, her canary, and it felt like home whenever we visited. There was only one bedroom, with a double bed, so my sister and I slept 'top to tail' in an old camp bed, with a crochet blanket and a hot-water bottle for extra warmth. Grandma was a big knitter. I would sit in front of the open fire with my back against the sofa and listen to the sound of her needles click-clacking. I was amazed that she could knit while she was watching TV and not even look at her hands. Her cooking was like a big hug, very meat and two veg – maybe pork chops, chips and peas with a generous helping of gravy, and baked apples for pudding.

She smoked Guards cigarettes; there were packets of them in every drawer in the flat, and she would rest a cigarette in her mouth, the ash growing. I sat, fascinated, waiting for it to drop, and just in time she would stop knitting and tap the cigarette into the little brass ashtray on the arm of the sofa. I remember years later, when I was a teenager, the government was due to announce a budget, and Grandma said if they put up the price of ciggies then she would quit smoking. They did put the price up and sure enough she never smoked another cigarette from that day. She didn't even mention it. You would never have known she had been a smoker.

When we did go home for the holidays, it felt awkward to start with while we settled back in with our parents, who felt a little bit like strangers. That didn't last long though, and we were soon a tight family unit of four again. We didn't need anyone else, although, frustratingly, Mum would try to hook us up with people of our own age, which resulted in uncomfortable play dates while the adults chatted and us children sized each other up.

I know this lifestyle may seem transient and discombobulating to some. There is a smallish part of me that wishes I had grown up in a rambling farmhouse in Dorset where my childhood bedroom would remain unchanged, with pop posters on the walls, gymkhana trophies on the shelves, my growing height marked on the doorframe, the family dog curled up on my bed and a view of a blossomy apple tree with a creaky swing. That sort of thing. I wonder what it would have been like to be rooted to one place, with the same group of friends, and years later to return to it with my own child and push him on my old swing. But then, how many of us can do that?

My early years may have looked unconventional to some, and I can see why, but I know how lucky I was. I had an incredible childhood, full of exotic adventure, independence and family. I didn't miss out; instead, I was enriched by it all. It instilled in me a sense of curiosity, an interest in different cultures and an empathy with others that has benefited me in my career and life.

It also taught me the importance of creating a home wherever I end up and how little I really need to enable that. Many of us have too much stuff. I find it fascinating that when we are asked the hypothetical (and admittedly dramatic) question of what we would rescue from our house in a fire, the most common response after 'people' and 'pets' is 'photographs'. What we really mean by that is memories, the most precious things of all. Now my mum is in an assisted living home around the corner from me, she has very few belongings, but what she does have carries great significance for her, and I can tell you the story associated with each of them.

I think I get my love of homemaking from my mum after watching her achieve it repeatedly over the years with apparent ease. She didn't always have much to work with, but as a child I didn't notice peeling wallpaper or unattractive decorative features because, like my grandma, Mum filled our home with warmth and love.

While houses are just bricks and mortar to me and I don't get emotionally attached to a property, I am a very good nest-builder. Even when I'm in a hotel room, I unpack immediately. I could have arrived at 3 a.m., but I still empty my bag, hang up clothes, line up beauty products in the bathroom and spritz the pillow with sleep spray. I can transform a space into my own and have the kettle on in minutes, like it's an Olympic sport. Perhaps it should be. I would be in line for a medal.

I am proud of being a homebird. My favourite type of day off is to potter around the house, tidying up, doing a little bit of cooking, drinking tea, reading the papers and enjoying the quiet after a busy week. It's my safe place, where I can be completely me, with no make-up and my bra off! On the flip side, I am a little territorial as I don't like my things being moved around, it unsettles me. I want to feel totally comfortable, and I want guests to relax the instant they walk through the door. When family and friends stay over, I make their bedroom an almost hotel-like experience, with dressing gowns, flowers, candles and even a travel kettle for those early risers, like my mum, who may want to make a cuppa and drink it in bed before the sun comes up.

Have you ever thought about what 'home' means to you? Is it where you were born? Where your parents are or where your children grew up? Maybe it's something you can't put your finger on or haven't found yet. Our definitions of it vary. For me, home truly is where the heart is. And where the dog is. Where I can be just as happy alone as I am with my loved ones. That's not about a building or even a location, it is a feeling I carry with me wherever I go. It's the foundation from which everything else flows: a superpower that can ground me whenever I need it most.

2

Good Girls Don't Get Expelled

I wasn't sent to boarding school – I chose to go, even though my parents thought I was too young and tried to talk me out of it. When I say boarding school, I need to explain the set-up because it wasn't what you might imagine. I wasn't shipped off to one of those all-girls jolly hockey sticks schools in the countryside where you were only allowed out to the village shop on a Saturday. I was in London, for a start.

The Royal Soldiers' Daughters' School was an independent girls' boarding school of royal patronage, founded in 1855 with buildings to match its age and grandeur. It was for army kids only, whose parents were spread out across the world. The place seemed ancient to me and incredibly spooky, with its great hall, creaky wooden floorboards, echoing cold dormitories and gloomy sanatorium. While we were there, we watched them building a new school within the grounds, which looked like a modern block of flats.

While it was technically called a 'school', we weren't actually taught there. Instead, we went to Hampstead Parochial primary school, which was a walk up Hampstead Hill, and while there must have been prefects around to keep an eye on us, I had a sense of independence and freedom every day on that walk.

I don't remember taking my 11-plus, the exam that determined what sort of secondary school I'd end up at. Julia would talk about going to the headmaster's office and being given a test to do, but I don't recall this. I think it's because nobody made a fuss, there was no build-up or stress around revision and no fear about what failure might mean. It was all very low key, so it didn't impact me.

I must have done something right because I passed and joined my sister at the all-girls Grey Coat Hospital grammar school in Westminster, which was down the road from the boys' school. Cue a lot of flirting! Even though the uniform held us back somewhat. In summer, we had to wear a blue and white spotty dress with a white Peter Pan collar, ankle socks, white gloves (not sensible for Tube travel) and regulation boaters, which we would try to squish in our bags. In the winter we were in actual heavy grey coats and felt bowler hats with a maroon band, and woe betide anyone who got caught without their hat on.

It was a very good school and while I may not have been an academic whizz-kid, I met my best friend Jennie on my first day at Grey Coat and made great friendships that I still have now.

Every afternoon, on the way back from school, we would meander slowly along Hampstead High Street looking for the local boys who used to hang around there. We did the same every Saturday when we were allowed out. It was all very innocent. We loved the excitement of it, but that was as far as it went.

Recently, we were in a *Loose Women* production meeting talking about a survey that had just come out focused on how parents find the school summer holidays difficult because of keeping their children entertained for six weeks. And I thought, really? Aren't kids allowed to be bored anymore? Just try sitting on a wall, kicking your heels for hours on end. Or lounging on a patch of grass with a pal and waiting for boys to walk past. Or roaming around the local area looking for boys we could walk past. Sometimes we would get word about where they could be and we would rush up to the top of the high street, only to find they had walked down the other side.

We never had any money. We just hung around. And if someone did have money, perhaps from a birthday, they would buy chips from the Wimpy, which the rest of us hoped to share. Or go to the Swiss chalet-style coffee house that had just opened in Hampstead. It had an outdoor café area, which we had never seen before, so it seemed quite sophisticated. It did the most amazing hot chocolate with whipped cream on top. Again, a new one on us. Two of us would sit down and order one drink and then the rest of us would swoop, like seagulls, so there could be six of us sitting around one hot chocolate.

Once we were a bit older, around fourteen, we were allowed out for longer with an evening curfew. Most Saturdays, Jennie and I would meet at Sloane Square and wander down the famous and trendy King's Road. Whenever I'm there now, I have such a strong sense of nostalgia and it brings back such great memories. I can see Jennie and me strutting down the road in platform shoes and flared jeans. It was the place to be.

We went to all the clothes shops and tried on stuff we had no intention of buying because we couldn't afford it. We mooched around the market full of seventies' fashion, including big platform boots. Then we would head to Boots to test every lip gloss, the roller-ball type, which was so sticky it looked like we'd been eating a jam doughnut and it had run down our chins. A quick spritz of a perfume tester and we were on our way.

There was a famous coffee shop there called Picasso, where lots of actors and rock stars used to go, and we would try to scrape together enough money to share a cappuccino (a coffee that was frothy? With chocolate powder sprinkled on top? Wow!) between us and hang around in the hope we could see a few famous people.

At school, I would skip meals so I could save up my dinner money and spend it on a pack of ten Consulate cigarettes, seduced by the advert showing a beautiful girl with long blonde hair in a white dress, stepping on stones across a babbling brook. The tagline was 'cool as a mountain stream' and I thought if I smoked, I might look like she did. It seemed so glamorous.

I had been keen to smoke from an early age. When I was about ten, my parents had popped around to the neighbours on the army base and my sister was in charge. She came into the sitting room to see me standing in front of the mirror, pretending to smoke one of Dad's cigarettes with a bottle of Mum's Babycham in the other hand.

'What on earth do you think you're doing?' Goody-Two-Shoes (Julia) squawked.

'Come and have a go!' I said, admiring my reflection. 'It's great!' That set the tone for my teenage years.

School was a sideline to my social life. I was an average student, but I messed around a lot and I wish I hadn't. I don't have many regrets in life because I think it's a pointless exercise, but I do look back and think I should have tried harder at school, and I would have done better. Instead, I did the bare minimum and thought I could still get the grades . . . big mistake.

I had just finished my O levels and the summer was stretching ahead of me. I wouldn't allow myself to think about results day, I was determined to enjoy the last couple of weeks in London before I went home for the school holiday. By this point, my dad had left the army and my parents had moved to Cawsand, a small fishing village near Plymouth. Without the army paying, my boarding school was unaffordable, but I had been granted a governors' bursary, which halved the cost and meant I could stay on for my A levels, so the next couple of years were mapped out for me.

It was Friday night, and I was out, as usual. We had a curfew, but I never took any notice of it and one of the younger girls would sneak down and unlock the back door at 10 p.m. for those who stayed out later. This particular evening, I arrived back and, panic-stricken, the girl on door duty said, 'Oh my God, Mrs Sibley knows you are out and she's on the warpath.' My heart was in my mouth. Shit, shit and triple shit! Mrs Sibley was the headmistress and not somebody I wanted to mess with.

I raced up the stairs as I could hear the staff lift coming up, skidded into the room I shared with two other girls and jumped, fully clothed, into bed. A second later, Mrs Sibley threw open the door, hit the light and shouted, 'Ruth Langsford!'

I proceeded to deliver one of the best performances of my life as I yawned, eyes squinting against the brightness, and pretended to surface out of a very deep sleep. Mrs Sibley marched over and pulled back the bed covers to reveal me still wearing my coat and shoes. 'I will see you in my office tomorrow morning,' she said, before turning on her heel and stomping out. I knew I would need to be very charming and apologetic, knowing it would blow over.

Sitting opposite her the next morning, I wore my best sorry face as Mrs Sibley went on for a bit about not setting a good example to the younger girls and I nodded along. Blah, blah, blah.

'Which is why,' she said, 'you will be going home this afternoon.'

'Oh, OK. What, for the weekend?' I said. That seemed like a bit of an overreaction, but I guess she wanted to make an example of me.

'No. For good, I'm afraid. The governors are not renewing your bursary. You won't be coming back.'

I had been at the boarding school since I was seven and I was now sixteen. It was a place of security and my home for a large part of my childhood. It also meant that if I was no longer allowed to board then I couldn't stay at Grey Coat school either. My entire life changed in an instant.

I was in shock. I left her office and went straight to the public phone box. I didn't call my parents because the headmistress had already spoken to them and I wasn't ready to face their wrath, so I called my best friend, Jennie.

'I've been expelled,' I sobbed.

'What do you mean? Aren't you coming back after the summer?' She was devastated. We didn't mention the fact that the school had tried to keep us apart because I was deemed a bad influence on her, my very clever friend.

Jennie met me at Victoria coach station where I was catching the bus home and we threw our arms around each other, wailing, declaring our undying love and promising to write (no mobile phones or texting in those days). Then I had to sit on a coach for hours, contemplating my fate. I had packed so quickly I'd left things behind including my loyal teddy, which I never got back. There was a metaphor for the end of my childhood, right there.

Dad collected me from Plymouth coach station. He was very quiet, which was the worst response ever. I was really close to him and couldn't bear the silent treatment.

'You've been a bit stupid, haven't you,' he said finally. So, this was the angle he was taking, and I had my retort ready.

'Yes, but you told me about all the things you used to get up to at school, and this really wasn't as bad.' I thought I was on safe ground with this argument.

'Maybe, but I never got caught, Ruthiee.' Dad used the affectionate double 'ee' nickname he always gave me. 'That's the point. You should have been smarter. Do you want to end up on the peanut counter in Woolworths?' This was a rhetorical question that he often asked, designed to shake me into thinking about my future. We were so alike, he and I, we clashed a lot because of it, but I know how much he regretted coasting through school, and he didn't want me to make the same mistake. He would be quite hard on me and then in the next breath recount some funny story about how badly behaved he had been at my age.

Mum met me at the door. 'I am so disappointed in you,' she said, looking disappointed. This was worse than the silent treatment. In that moment, the years of schoolgirl jinks, all the 'oh I'm quite a laugh' or 'I stay out late and never get caught' and 'I walk around Hampstead with the boys' felt silly. I wasn't too cool for school and my cockiness evaporated instantly.

That night, I got into bed, in a room that didn't really feel like mine, in a house I didn't know, and I gave myself a stiff talking to. What an absolute idiot I had been and now here I was, stuck in a bloody fishing village in Cornwall where I didn't know anybody. All my friends were in London, and I wasn't going back. Added to this, Mum could barely look at me and Dad was frustrated that, while I had turned out like him, I hadn't been as good at being bad.

Why couldn't I be more like my sister? She had aced all her exams and just finished her A levels. She had been head girl at the Royal Soldiers and deputy head girl at Grey Coat, for goodness' sake. She would never have been thrown out. I now wish I'd been expelled for something a bit more dramatic, worthy of retelling over the years, like getting caught snogging on school premises or setting fire to the dormitory with a lit cigarette.

It felt like my life was a disaster and I had only lived sixteen years of it, but more bad news was yet to come because my O level results were pending.

Back in the day, results would arrive from the school in the post in a self-addressed envelope, and there was no mistaking my own handwriting. Every morning of those first days back at home, I would jump out of bed early so I could get to the post before anyone else, which is quite some feat for a teenager! I hadn't done any revision and didn't even finish my maths paper, so I knew it would be terrible, but this was exactly the wrong time for my parents to find out. I needed to get to the letter first.

Then, one morning, there it was, the envelope written in my own hand, and Mum called from the kitchen, 'Is that the post? Have your results arrived?' And I shouted back, 'No, not yet!' I shoved the envelope in my dressing-gown pocket and ran upstairs to my bedroom. In a cold sweat, I opened it, and it was even worse than I had thought. I had only passed four subjects and one of those was needlework. Three subjects, including maths, were ungraded: a fail with bells on!

I came back downstairs in tears. I had decided the best course of action was honesty with a lot of embellishment. I was really good at drama at school and so I went for the outraged injustice approach.

'Mum, I did just get my results, and I can't believe it. They are really bad . . .'

'Oh darling, I'm sure they can't be that awful,' she reassured me.

'No, they really are, and I just don't understand it because I worked so, so hard,' I wailed, handing the slip over to her. She read it and paused.

'Oh. Well, you got English,' she said encouragingly.

Dad saw straight through me. 'You can't have worked hard because if you had done you would have passed them all. Anyway, there you go. That's what you get for messing around. So, looks like it's going to be the peanut counter in Woolworths for you after all then, Ruthiee.'

A feeling of doom settled over me. Both my parents looked at me and said in unison, 'So what are you going to do now?'

What was I going to do now?! If only I had someone to talk to. I hadn't made any friends locally. There was a group of teenagers from the village who would come and sit on the wall overlooking the beach, below our house. I sat in the window seat and spied on them, hiding behind the curtain if they looked up in my direction. Then the inevitable moment when I came back from the shops one day and there they all were. 'All right?' they said. 'Oh yeah, hello,' I mumbled back, going bright red and running up to the house. I felt like an alien in my London look of Levi jeans tucked into cowboy boots, wearing Dad's old shirts with the collars cut off.

I got into sixth form at Saltash comprehensive school to study A levels despite my results, and while I still didn't have a focused attitude around education, my work ethic was strong if it involved cold, hard cash. The first summer home I worked in a beach café, where I was a bit scared of my boss, a tough but great businesswoman. I had to take orders and carry trays of tea and cake down to the customers on the beach, trundling carefully across the pebbles.

I told Mum I had a job. 'Oh, that's fantastic, Ruth. So how much do you want to give towards housekeeping?'

'Sorry, housekeeping?'

'Yes.' Mum was firm. 'Now you're working, you can contribute to the household.'

I was so shocked, but she meant it, and we worked out a percentage I could pay her weekly towards bills. I look back on this now and am grateful that she instilled this in me, although I liked to give a boundary a prod and was often negotiating with her about when I would pay and if I could owe her because there was a pair of jeans I really, really wanted to buy. My wages would be spent before I'd earned them. Mum would always let me off the hook if I promised to pay her back, although we joke that I probably still owe her five quid!

School took a back seat; again, I did no work. The jobs are more what I remember. In my second summer, I got a job down the road at the Criterion Hotel, which was run by the absolutely delightful husband-and-wife team Mr and Mrs Shimell. I was a waitress in the restaurant, and at the end of my first morning shift, as I was clearing the tables, Mr Shimell called up to me from the kitchen at the bottom of the big stone staircase: 'Breakfast is ready!' I was nonplussed and went down to discover the staff sitting around the table, while Mrs Shimell cooked us eggs and bacon and Mr Shimell served us. This happened every morning. They looked after us so well, were so kind to us, and as a consequence we would have gone to the ends of the earth for them.

Once a diner was incredibly rude to me because the Dover sole was off the menu and Mr Shimell stepped in and quietly asked him to leave. 'Nobody speaks to my staff like that.' What a legend. Mrs Shimell was a superb baker and sent me off at the end of my afternoon shift with slices of leftover coffee and walnut or Victoria sandwich cake. I worked there for a couple of years, and I have never forgotten them, nor the way they treated their team, with such respect and care it earned them our deep loyalty in return.

I worked there every Saturday before racing home to get changed and then going out on the town to blow my wages. That would have been either a ferry then a bus to Plymouth to go to the Fiesta Suite nightclub, Diamond Lil's or the Roxy on the renowned Union Street, where they played soul music, which I loved, and then a taxi back. Or we (by now, I had a good group of local friends) would stay in the village and wander between the five pubs because everyone turned a blind eye to under-age drinking in those days.

It didn't leave much time for studying, particularly not when I would bunk off to mooch around Saltash high street and sit in the bakery, drinking coffee and smoking. I failed economics and politics A levels, managing to pass English. So ended my disastrous educational career.

With the benefit of fifty years of hindsight, I can see how stupid it was to mess about at school and not achieve what I was capable of. That said, I don't believe anyone means to chuck their education away. Yes, I may have thrown my qualifications away, but I think I absorbed more of the teaching than I realised. I didn't make the most of my school journey, but it wasn't a complete waste of time either. I am not here to advocate messing around and flunking school as a surefire way to ultimate success, but exams are not the be-all and end-all of life.

Not everyone can be a chemist. Or a lawyer. Or an accountant. It isn't just about academic achievements; it's about knowing what you want to do with the rest of your life. That can be an impossible question to answer. Particularly when you are fourteen and choosing GCSE subjects with no idea where you are heading. I look at kids now and think there's too much pressure heaped on them around exams and grades. And then the expectation they will go to university and come out with a degree. This seems to be shifting as more young people see the benefit in getting out in the workplace or taking on an apprenticeship.

A great number of people I meet don't do a job associated with their degree, often finding their way to where they want to be via a strange and unplottable route. I found this fascinating and helpful when I was trying to guide my son, Jack, and I would say to him, sometimes a degree is just about showing a level of learning and retention, which can give you confidence in many jobs, not just the subject you are studying.

Full disclosure: I didn't tell Jack how limited my qualifications were when he went through GCSEs and A levels. I remembered my dad regaling me with his stories of getting up to no good at school and how I thought I could behave the same way. I didn't want Jack to make the same mistake, so I gave him the impression that I'd done rather well. On one occasion, sitting with him while he was doing his politics homework, he asked me to read something through and I told him where I thought it was wrong. He disagreed. I knew I was right. We went back and forth about it until I said, 'Jack, which one of us has got politics A level?' To which he responded, 'You?' And I said, 'Exactly, so please listen to me.' I don't have politics A level, but he did listen to me.

My worry was that Jack might think he could coast his exams because I had and look where I'd ended up, doing a job I loved. I didn't want him to drop the ball for a single second, particularly not in today's competitive world.

I haven't done too badly, all things considered, but it was sheer luck that I got on the telly and then it was hard work, grit and determination that kept me there. Sometimes it's about someone seeing your potential and being prepared to champion you, which is exactly what happened to me. And in return, I have done the same and paid that forward, helping out if someone is deserving but maybe a little lost. I know how powerful it is for someone on a higher rung of the career ladder to see you and offer to help in some small way, and I try to do the same whenever I can.

All of this said and done – and to contradict myself a little (because we are allowed to think two different things at the same time) – having decent results is the ideal scenario. That was my attitude with Jack. It sets you off in the right direction and it can make you more self-reliant too. Whatever happens, we need to remember it is never too late to do something new or fulfil a long-held dream, although I think it's unlikely I will become a professional ballet dancer or an accountant!

3
What's the Worst That Can Happen?

In a career that has spanned over four (gulp) decades, with the majority of those years spent in live television, I have had my fair share of tricky situations and nail-biting, seat-of-my-pants moments. There are two that stay with me; the first was far back in the mists of time and the second was more recent and involved a lot of fake tan and sequins, which I write about in a few chapters' time. Let's go back to the almost beginning.

There I was, with a handful of paltry exam results and no clue what I wanted to do with the rest of my life. Why couldn't I be one of those impressive teenagers who knew exactly where they were heading? Because I was directionless. Enter Mum. Who suggested I do what she had done many years before and take a shorthand and typing course; and as I couldn't think of a good reason not to, or felt I was in no position to argue, I enrolled at Devonport College and discovered I quite liked it. More to the point, I was pretty good at it. I can still touch-type now, although I am a little heavy-handed on the keyboard because I was taught on a clunky manual typewriter with a carriage return (if you know, you know).

Around this time, I met a fantastic woman, Pat Savage, in our village pub. I would often bump into Pat and really liked chatting to her. She was PA to the Head of Presentation at our regional ITV station, Westward Television. One night she was asking me what plans I had for the future, and I was telling her how I didn't have a clue, how disappointed my parents were in me and that I was hoping secretarial qualifications would get me a temping job. Pat was sympathetic to my problem.

'Let me see if I can get you a meeting with our Head of Personnel at Westward TV, they are often looking for office staff,' she said supportively, and she was true to her word.

Pat's colleague Crispin invited me in for a chat on her recommendation and although he could see my questionable school grades, I think my personality and general keenness shone through. He said to carry on with my secretarial course and get in touch if and when I qualified. I had three months left of the nine-month course and every few weeks I would ring Crispin, just to check in, and he would say the same thing: 'Finish your course and we will talk.'

I passed with flying colours, the first time I had been a success at anything, which was such a good and unfamiliar feeling. I rang Crispin immediately. There were no jobs, but he promised he would be in touch as soon as something came up. In the meantime, I got a job covering maternity leave in the typing pool at Devon and Cornwall County Council, which was not where I had imagined the eighteen-year-old me would end up. I was with the loveliest group of women who were so welcoming to me, but as a junior I found the work repetitive. There was a table in the middle of the room, with an in-tray and an out-tray. I had to take a piece of work from the in-tray, type it up and put it in the out-tray. I did this for hours and hours and hours, with a lot of audio-typing thrown in.

I had never thought in terms of a career, just how to earn money, but this made me wonder if I needed a different approach. As luck would have it, Crispin got back in touch and asked me if I would be interested in having an interview for a transmission loggist job. A what?! I had no idea what one of those did, but I didn't care if it got me out of the typing pool. So, I said yes.

I found myself in the smart boardroom at Westward TV, sitting opposite David Sunderland, the Head of Presentation. David was the top dog, in charge of everything that was presented on screen, but I was too young and inexperienced to be scared so I didn't overthink it. We chatted and he took me down to the control room to show me around, and left me there to take it all in.

The moment I walked into that control room, I knew. This was where I wanted to be for the rest of my life, in this dark space with banks of monitors, a huge desk with lots of buttons and a busy team of people. They were mostly men, of course, but there was one woman, who was telling a continuity presenter behind a glass panel that 'we are coming to you in 10 . . . 9 . . . 8'. She seemed to be doing lots of timings on a machine and complicated sums before counting down to *Coronation Street*, a show we all watched as a family. I absorbed everything.

David asked me when I could start. I couldn't believe I had got the job and was thrilled, even though I wasn't sure what it was – the detail didn't matter. My immediate excitement was then followed by the chilling fear that if I was the person responsible for adding up timings, I would need to be confident with numbers. Did David know I had failed my maths O level? There was no point panicking because I started a week later so there was nothing I could do about that, other than try damn hard. My typing-pool colleagues were all lovely to me and waved me off with flowers and cake.

I started in the presentation office, preparing and typing up running schedules, and was only needed in the control room to cover meal breaks and illness. It was a good way for someone so young and inexperienced to be eased in, plus I was there during Westward's regional television heyday, which made it fun, interesting and well paid. I met one of my best friends, Sam, in the office and we still love to reminisce about those days when we get together.

It wasn't long before I was moved into the gallery and control room full time. I had been hoping for a job there and it felt like a dream come true, I was so happy. I worked with the continuity presenters in their little studio behind the glass panel, where they operated their own camera and lights. They wrote their own scripts and there was no autocue. My job was to count them in and out, as we switched from local programming to network shows and then back again. Time would be gained and lost depending on what was going on, so I had to carefully monitor and communicate this. For a girl who was hopeless with numbers, I was a dab hand at working out minutes and seconds. Maybe using maths in a practical setting that made sense to me had been the answer all along.

The continuity presenters were not just delivering voice-overs, they were in vision too, and on Saturday nights the men wore black tie. It was the early 1980s – think Jilly Cooper's *Rivals*, which perfectly captured the world of franchise telly through the misogynist lens of that time. I was the girl in the gallery, in a male-dominated environment, who, as well as doing my job, was also in charge of taking food orders, doing the tea run and getting snacks for the guys. Why was that?! Why were women expected to sort out catering for the men when we were all working as hard as each other?

Women had to deal with sexist remarks and flirty banter on a regular basis, and we were expected to laugh it off, which we did – but I remember us being feisty and standing up for ourselves when we needed to. Someone once patted my backside, and he got a sharp elbow from me. He never did it again. Then there was the stationery store, where I would go and pick up supplies for the department, only to be confronted with posters and calendars of naked women plastered on the walls – something that, thankfully, wouldn't be allowed these days. The eighties was a different time and thank goodness so much has changed over the years, enabling women to now challenge inappropriate language and behaviour, although there is still much work to be done.

After a few happy years, I began to think about what might be next and had an idea to find out more about being a floor manager because it involved elements of my current job and appealed to the organiser in me. That felt like a good plan, but there were other plans afoot that I knew nothing about.

I was in the control room one Friday and I got a call from my boss, David Sunderland, asking me to pop up to his office. I grabbed my shorthand pad because I assumed he was going to give me a task. Ever the professional.

'Ah Ruth, we need to find a holiday relief continuity presenter. It's not a full-time job . . .' I began to make a note of this, assuming he wanted me to put out an advert somewhere. 'And I wondered if you fancied having an audition for it?' I did a double take, expecting someone to have walked in behind me, but he was looking straight at me.

'What, me?' I said. I had never shown any interest in being on screen or asked to be considered.

'I dunno.' He was smiling. 'I just thought you might be quite good. Anyway, no need to give me an answer now. Think about it over the weekend and let me know on Monday.'

I came out of David's office in a daze and headed straight to the payphone (remember those?!) in the corridor to call home. Dad answered and I told him what had just happened and asked what he thought I should do about it.

'Oh, that's great, love,' he said, 'and don't worry about not having any experience. Just go for the audition and you will either get it or you won't. I mean, what's the worst that can happen?' That was my dad, glass more than half full. Had my mum picked up the phone, she probably would have given me all the reasons why I shouldn't risk it because she was more cautious than Dad. I wasn't leaving my old job, I was just adding another skill to my CV, so if it didn't work out then it didn't matter because there was no risk involved. Other than a dented ego, but I wasn't worried about that. After all, Dad was right, what was the worst that could happen?

What's the Worst That Can Happen?

On Monday I told David I would like to audition, which involved presenting a news bulletin, voicing three commercials and talking for ninety seconds about myself, which was the hardest bit. As people found out I was being considered for the role, I sensed discomfort. I could have been wrong, but it felt like there was an assumption about me being an ambitious typist and I wanted to explain to everyone that while I hadn't asked for this, it was an opportunity I couldn't pass up. I think some of my colleagues didn't expect me to get the job, but I did and with it came a heavy dose of imposter syndrome, which I had not experienced before. Whether people were talking about me or not didn't matter because I felt nervous and insecure, and I was convinced they must be. What was I thinking? How on earth could I be on TV?

The theory was that I would continue as a transmission assistant and switch to continuity presenting to cover holidays. I had done two days' training with the suave, debonair Roger and on the third day there was a phone call. Roger was ill and wouldn't be coming in. They rang round every other announcer, but it was early in the morning, and nobody was picking up, so all eyes turned to me. Looked like they had no choice and neither did I.

I was absolutely terrified. This was not how I wanted my screen debut to go, there was still so much to learn, but there was nobody else available. I was sent into make-up while they made a last-ditch attempt to find a professional before giving up and accepting their fate and mine. I was thrust on to live television. Luckily, I was well versed in the timings and structure of the announcements, and I knew what ten seconds felt like (although this can feel like an eternity on live telly), but this was a baptism of raging fire. My mouth went dry, and I thought, I can't do this. Maybe I'll throw up or pass out, or both, and then how will that look on live telly? But I didn't, I kept going and then it was over in a blur. I had done my first broadcast and couldn't remember a moment of it.

I loved being a transmission assistant so I wasn't hankering to get back into the studio after that first hair-raising experience, and I was eased in carefully after that, little things here and there. By the time I was offered a full-time continuity presenter role, I was ready. I would get stopped when I was shopping in Plymouth and people would talk fondly about how nervous I had been to begin with.

'Oh, bless her, dear of her, you're much better now! Isn't she, Derek? We were only saying how comfortable you are now, weren't we, Derek?!' The West Country dialect uses 'dear of her' as an expression of sympathetic affection, which summed up how much the local audience seemed to be rooting for me. I say that London is the place I have spent the longest time and feels most like home, but I was very much part of the south-west community during the years I lived there. Plymouth was a second home for me.

As well as the general public, my friend Ian Stirling, a seasoned continuity presenter, gave me a lot of helpful and honest feedback. He would call me and say 'Stop wobbling your head', something I still do when I am really nervous. Or he would tell me off for saying 'absolutely' too often and I would say 'I don't!' and he would say 'You bloody well do!'. I found it remarkably easy to chat to camera. Ian would tell me to think of a family at home – maybe parents, a couple of kids, a grandma and a dog – and imagine I was talking just to them. Not the millions of unseen faces. Just one family settled in their cosy sitting room. It totally worked. He was the pal I needed, and his care and attention made me better in my role.

I was moved to the newsroom because I was good at reading the bulletins, but I found the newshound part of the job very stressful and hated having to go out in search of stories. I believe in showing vulnerability and asking for help if you don't know something and so I did that, and consequently had a lot of support during that time. People were there to teach me, and I wanted to learn. I was not a natural leader, I preferred to be part of a team, inspired by other people's energy and ideas, which I always gave them full credit for.

Ken MacLeod was the legendary news anchorman who had my total respect. He had been there years, was brilliant and also very kind to me. I was co-presenting the flagship six o'clock news show with him when I had my first studio interview, with a beauty queen guest. It was only a five-minute chat, so I had put together about five or six questions to ask her. I could feel the nerves rising but I knew I was prepared. What I wasn't ready for were her one-word answers, which meant I quickly ran out of questions and still had three minutes to fill. My mouth went dry, my mind went blank, and I turned to the news desk and squeaked, 'Back to you, Ken.' The cameras flew from me back to him in a panic. I was too inexperienced to fill in the time or realise I had all three cameras at that point, so I had just bailed and dropped everyone in it. It was a big lesson for every interview that has followed, and I always have more questions than it is ever possible to ask.

I was mortified and desperately apologetic afterwards, but Ken understood. He was so calm, nothing fazed him. 'Don't worry about it, darling. These things happen.' If the world was about to end in three minutes, he is the man you would want to break the news to you. The editor was a different story. He bawled me out in his glass-fronted office in the middle of the newsroom while everyone else pretended not to notice. I was determined not to cry until I got out of there and went straight to the toilet, where I could sob in private. Little did I know it wouldn't be long before I would be back in continuity, my favourite place.

It was 1992 and franchises across the network were up for renewal, including ours. The programme controller at South West (TSW) decided he wanted his faces of the station to be a regular presence in profile roles and he wanted me to go back to continuity and be the weekend presenter. I was thrilled. It was where I had started my broadcast journey and it was home for me, so I was delighted to go back.

I was in my stride, had all my notes, wrote my scripts, managed the new autocue and was not fazed by any technical issues. I have a slightly photographic memory, which means I can see things on the page and they stick in my head. This job really was the best training for a career in live television.

The announcement of the winning bidder for the franchise was made on the day of my grandmother's funeral, so I had no idea what was happening. My then boyfriend met me at the crematorium and told me South West (TSW) had lost to West Country Television. This was a shock result for us all and it meant that I was suddenly catapulted into the freelance world.

I always say I wouldn't have got into presenting if it wasn't for my dad encouraging me to go for the audition, but the fact is, I wouldn't have been in telly in the first place if it hadn't been for my mum pushing me into the secretarial course. I credit them both for the direction my career took. In a life of sliding doors moments, this was a significant junction, and with their guidance I made my choice and I didn't look back. This has been a recurring theme for me when I have been faced with decisions and challenges, and I take gambles and try not to carry any regrets. As Dad always said, 'Ruthiee, what's the worst that can happen?' and this has stood me in good stead. I recommend you keep this question up your sleeve for those times when you may need it.

4

Imposter Syndrome

So, there I was, reeling from the news that TSW had lost the franchise we were all certain would be theirs, and staring straight into the cruel face of redundancy. In that moment, I imagined myself back in the typing pool. I knew I wouldn't be out of work for long because of my secretarial qualifications, but I also knew I had a foothold in a career that I absolutely loved. What could I do to keep myself in the TV industry?

I needn't have worried because West Country Television, the company that had won the franchise, offered me a presenting job almost immediately. So OK, it was to present a business programme, and I was likely one of the most unqualified people to have been given this, but at least my enthusiasm was admirable. It was made by the independent production company Two Four Productions, founded by two guys – Charles Wace and Christopher Slade – who worked incredibly hard and took the company from something small to the huge success it is today. I was grateful to them for their offer of work, and it kept me on screen while I began to put myself out in the freelance presenting world.

I started to pick up more on-screen work on programmes like BBC's *Countryfile* and I realised quite quickly that being a freelancer in Plymouth was going to be almost impossible when most of the telly jobs were in London, so I took the plunge and moved back up there. Considering how much I didn't want to live in the West Country when I was sixteen, I missed being there, but I knew being back in the city was a chance to keep my fledgling career on track.

I was pretty clueless about how it all worked because I had been in a staff job for much of my working life. I remember being infuriated with the BBC because they hadn't paid me and I mentioned it to a telly friend, who was angry on my behalf and wanted to know when I had invoiced them. Invoiced them? I didn't know what she meant. I had done the work and now I was waiting for a payment, so what did an invoice have to do with it? She sat me down, gave me a template and talked me through what I had to do, including charging for the expenses I had incurred. Train ticket? Hotel? Lunch? And where were my receipts? I began to feel pretty stupid! It was a big learning curve.

When I first met my (now ex-) husband, Eamonn Holmes, he remembered me from an episode of *Countryfile*. I mentioned working for the programme and he asked if I had done a filming segment on Rathlin Island, off the coast of Northern Ireland.

'Did you do a piece to camera in the back of a boat? You were wearing a red shirt?' he said, and I nodded, surprised by his memory. 'I hadn't seen you on screen before and I thought you were very good.' As chat-up lines go, it was a pretty successful one.

I remembered that day too because I hate boats and the crossing was really rough. I was panicking but I didn't want to appear unprofessional, and besides, I needed the money, so I plastered on a smile and did a piece to camera while the boat pitched from side to side. This also led to more work.

One Sunday afternoon I was at friends for lunch, and I met David Pritchard, who was the producer for the infamous chef Keith Floyd. We got chatting and he said he would love to work with me, which was a big accolade. He came up with an idea entitled *Brief Encounters*, which was a type of travel show with me going around the West Country meeting interesting people who were doing weird and wonderful things. I played underwater hockey, was hoisted into a tree to listen to the dawn chorus and dressed up as a cowboy to join a re-enactment group. Just a few of the madcap things I got involved in. We made two series, and I had such fun working with David. He was one of those creative geniuses who really understood the medium of television and what the audience wanted.

I didn't like being freelance then and I still don't, it's not a natural state of being for me. I would love a full-time job where my tax is already sorted out, and I don't have to worry about my future. Considering how long I have worked in television and how few staff jobs are available, it's interesting that I still find the lack of security hard to deal with. I am constantly looking ahead and considering what the next job may be, even when I'm happily ensconced in a year's contract.

The upside of this is that I am not complacent. Telly is a notoriously fickle place to be, and I have fallen foul of it several times in my career, but it keeps me on my toes. My long-term future is uncertain, but then isn't that the case for so many of us these days, no matter what industry we work in? The reality is I have never been out of work for more than a couple of weeks, other than on one occasion. I was presenting the BBC's *The Really Useful Show* in 1998, a daytime consumer programme that I loved doing because it was live, there was a big team, a daily phone-in and we covered such varied, interesting and helpful subjects. You could almost call it a public service. I was convinced it would be recommissioned because everyone was really pleased with it and the ratings were great, but a new programme controller arrived and scrapped it. I had just bought a little house in London, and I thought, how the hell am I going to pay my mortgage?

That was the longest period I was without work, and I sent showreels out and hoped every phone call would be my agent on the other end with an offer of work. My CV showed a list of TV credits with a journalistic theme, which was entirely reflective of my career to date.

I wasn't a trained journalist; in the TSW newsroom, I had been learning on the job. Yes, I sat in front of the camera to present the six o'clock news every night and turned out to be a good newsreader, but the bosses didn't know what to do with me during the day, so they pushed me into becoming a journalist before I went back into continuity. This had done nothing for my confidence and my imposter syndrome returned with a vengeance. I worked hard to ignore the judgemental voice in my head, but it never went away. I was not in my natural environment and was uncomfortable with the blokey bluster and relentless deadlines.

When I was there, I was sent out to cover news stories, which was like being thrown into the lion's den. Like the time they sent me out on a serious assault story, for which I was wholly ill-equipped and relied on the brilliant camera crew to help me through it. Coupled with this were all the trained journalists who were asking 'who the hell is this girl?' behind my back, so I knew I had a lot to prove. I don't feel like that now. I may not have a degree in journalism or have worked my way up through several different newsrooms, but my practical experience has proved invaluable. I have a journalistic head for interviews, which is useful in my job. Couple that with a natural curiosity about people and I know I am good at what I do, but I haven't always found it easy to be so self-assured.

It took me a long time to truly believe in myself and now I have utter confidence in my journalism skills. Would I want to work on a news programme? No. It's not my bag. Do I love interviewing people? Absolutely. This is my natural home.

It's a skill to interview someone, particularly those who haven't been on television before or are nervous or about to talk about the worst time of their life. I want them to feel secure and safe with me and this begins before the cameras start rolling. It's the moment we meet, either in the green room or the studio, and the conversation we have. I want people to trust me enough to share their story and be able to speak freely, which is hard to achieve in an alien environment like a TV studio. Just before we go on air, I reassure them that we are just having a conversation, and while we are live I hope I show them I am really listening to what they are saying. The trick is to manage this while the gallery are giving me a hard count in my earpiece. Knowing we have ten seconds to a break and tying up the chat in that time is an ability I'm proud of. I get that it's not very transferable in other industries but it's imperative in live telly!

I was a guest on something recently and I was completely at sea without my earpiece. It really threw me. I'm used to knowing what is going on and where we are timing-wise with the programme. I worry that I'll be talking too much, and I wonder what the count is. I'm definitely better in the control seat.

Back when I started out, I'm not sure the term 'imposter syndrome' even existed. We thought of it more as a lack of confidence in a position we had been entrusted with, but I like the concept of the imposter because that is exactly what it felt like. I could be found out at any moment.

It didn't disappear overnight for me. It was a gradual realisation that it was holding me back in situations that I shouldn't be worrying about. Imposter syndrome is sneaky and likes to chip away at our belief in ourselves, appearing to target women more than men, but I know it isn't gender-specific. I would sometimes say I wasn't a journalist because I didn't have a degree in it or have all the relevant experience, and Eamonn would tell me to stop saying I wasn't because I was.

Then there were times when I managed to silence my inner doubts completely, like when I was approached by *This Morning* in the late nineties. It was a show I'd loved from the early days of Richard and Judy, so when my agent called me to say two ITV executives wanted to meet me to talk about a possible presenting role, I couldn't quite believe my ears. It was all a bit vague, but I didn't care. I got up early to meet them for breakfast at the Savoy, of all places. Such a grand, beautiful hotel set in an iconic building overlooking the River Thames. I felt a buzz of excitement and hope as I walked through the doors.

The two men swore me to secrecy, and I was intrigued. Richard and Judy were keen to reduce their commitment from five days to four, and the producers were looking for presenters to put together as a duo to present the show every Friday.

'Look no further,' I said, as this was not a time to play hard to get, 'because I am your girl.'

'Well, it's good to hear of your interest, but we are considering other people . . .' one of the men said.

'Please don't consider anyone else! I am your biggest fan. I've been watching the show for years.' I probably should have stopped talking, but I wanted to show how much this opportunity meant to me. I wasn't just a presenter for hire, I loved the programme, it was my dream to be on it. The magazine format appealed to me, and the way it managed to encompass so many different things in a two-hour slot. I didn't hold back, I was literally begging, which I don't recommend, but there we are.

I didn't get the job. They gave it to Fern Britton, who was brilliant, and it hurt less knowing someone great had beaten me to it, although I was still absolutely gutted. Fern began presenting every Friday morning, with John Leslie, and I thought my chance had passed until ITV got back in touch. Fern wanted to take school holidays off and only do Fridays in term time because she had young children, so would I step in as holiday cover? You bet I would. My memory is a bit murky on what happened next, but Richard and Judy decided to leave, Fern and John were promoted to the main show, and I was given the full-time Friday slot.

Funnily enough, I never once had imposter syndrome while I was working on *This Morning*. I think this was because I felt very at home there, among the topics I was discussing and the people I was working with. However, here is the thing about imposter syndrome: it can remain dormant for long periods of time and it likes to hide in the shadows. When it reappears, it helps if you recognise it for what it is, name it and openly talk about how you feel, because if you do it begins to shrink. I would talk to close friends and family about how I felt, and this really helped. It was also powerful to reassert my abilities and remind myself of my producer skills, creative flair and good old common sense, because our qualities are easy to undermine or forget. I didn't say this to anyone else but just in my head. I could have said it to myself in the mirror every morning, but I think people only do that in movies.

These days, we are encouraged to reframe these situations and see failure as a way to learn and grow. There is a language to use, jokes to be made and a lot written about dealing with imposter syndrome, which makes it relatable and also seem like something you can tackle in an afternoon. Of course, we know that isn't the case, but I'm glad we are calling it out in whatever way we can – and something tells me it may be less of an issue in the future.

5

Maybe Baby

There was an assumption among my family and friends that I was a career girl, which was true in part, because I loved my job, but they thought I had made it my priority in life. They didn't think I was bothered about having a family of my own. My sister, Julia, brought it up once and I said, 'Don't you think I would rather be you, with a husband and child? It's not that I don't want it. It's just that it hasn't happened for me yet. I haven't met the right person.'

And then I did meet the right person, and he had three children. Eamonn had separated from his wife but was still a very present father and I was concerned that he might not want more children. I would have understood if he hadn't. I was thirty-six and yet to hear the biological clock ticking, but I knew that he was the person I wanted to be with, so I brought up the subject very early on in our relationship. Eamonn knew how I felt. It wasn't his plan to have more children, but he loved me and wanted me to be happy. We both agreed we were open to it one day but were in no rush.

This was the first time I had talked to a partner about starting a family. In my previous relationships, a long-term commitment hadn't felt right for all sorts of reasons. I was either too young, not interested in having kids or knew I wasn't with the right person. If you lined up my ex-boyfriends (in what would be a relatively short line!), you would see that I definitely didn't have a type either. While I could imagine getting married and having children at some point in the future, that future felt very far away and I wasn't the sort of girl who daydreamed about being a bride or planned my perfect wedding dress.

At forty-one years old, I was thrilled to discover that I had fallen pregnant naturally. It felt like an absolute blessing considering the statistics for someone my age, which were stacked against me. We had been trying for six months and the worry began to creep in, so I decided if nothing had happened by the following month, I would see the doctor, but I didn't need to because I fell pregnant. I knew how lucky I was, when there were so many women who were struggling to conceive and going through IVF.

By this point, Eamonn and I had been together nearly six years, and I had got to know his children very well, with their mother's approval. She was instrumental in helping tell them about the new baby, so they didn't feel pushed out. Eamonn and I were not married at this point; in fact, we didn't tie the knot until Jack was eight. For me, the biggest commitment we could make to each other was to have a child together and we didn't need a wedding to prove that.

I enjoyed being pregnant. I didn't relish my body changing and my boobs were huge, but I was so excited that something I thought might not happen for me was about to. Other than the usual tiredness, I had no challenging symptoms and I continued to work on TV throughout my pregnancy, for *Loose Women* and as a guest presenter on *This Morning*, as well as a studio-based travel show. I still managed to get to antenatal classes. I remember at the first one a woman walked in, and I thought she was the teacher because she was really slim with no sign of a baby, whereas I was already big. In fact, I was so large, my doctor had to double-check I'd got my dates right! The woman sat next to me, and it turned out her baby was due around the same time as mine. I looked at her and thought, good God, am I having an elephant? Which turned out not to be the case, because Jack came out an average-size baby.

The woman who ran the antenatal classes had been doing it for years and was wonderful, very calm and sensible, which is exactly what you need as a first-time mum. One of the things she said was that while it was great to fill out a birth plan and write down how we wanted our labours to go, the baby would decide how it would be born and that may not be a water birth surrounded by whale music and candles. She told us to try to go with the flow.

It was a couple of weeks before the baby's due date and I was feeling a little unsettled. It was about 9 p.m. and I decided to go to bed, leaving Eamonn watching TV. I read my book for a bit, but I couldn't get comfortable, and I didn't feel the slightest bit tired, so I got up and went back downstairs, just as Eamonn was turning the lights out and coming to bed. He gave me a look and asked if I was OK, like he had a spidey sense of what was coming. 'Fine,' I said, 'I just can't sleep so I'm going to do a few emails and will come back up in a bit.'

There was no WhatsApp in those days, so we relied on group emails, and I sent the other women from the antenatal class a message asking if anyone else was still up. I cleaned the fridge. Then I found myself under the kitchen sink, clearing out an area that I would usually ignore. There I was at 1 a.m., heavily pregnant, Marigold gloves on, scrubbing the cupboard, when the words from my antenatal teacher popped into my head. 'Sometimes, just before labour, you may find yourself sorting out the airing cupboard or tidying a random space. We call this nesting.' It was like a lightbulb moment. I thought, is this it?

As I stood up, I felt a dull ache in my stomach, but I didn't think much of it. Even when that pain came again and I had to lean on the kitchen worktop until it passed. Eamonn appeared in his dressing gown. He was on GMTV in those days, which meant 4 a.m. starts, and he had woken to find that I was not in bed. 'I'm OK,' I said, 'just cramps. I think this is Braxton Hicks.' I didn't want to be the geriatric mother who immediately panicked and rushed to hospital at the slightest twinge. Eamonn felt differently, he was sure I was in the early stages of labour, and he was bemused by my reaction. He rang work to say he couldn't come in, even though I was telling him I was fine and he should go. It felt like a massive overreaction. That was until I called my lovely midwife, Maria.

I told her I had been up all night cleaning and that the pain was getting a little stronger, so she wanted to know how far apart the niggly spasms were. I wasn't really sure, maybe five minutes or so, and there was a pause and then she said, 'Ruth, why don't you head to the hospital? I am there today anyway so I will come and find you. It can't hurt to take a look.'

Eamonn rang my mum to let her know that I might be in labour. I was still in denial and had gone off to have a shower and wash my hair. I was absolutely not going to have this baby unless I had clean, blow-dried hair. By the time I got in the car, the pain was a series of undeniable contractions, and I had one that stopped me in my tracks. I couldn't move, it was so painful. Eamonn looked pale behind the wheel, convinced I was going to give birth in the car.

By 8 a.m., I was at the hospital and taken straight to a birthing room. Labour began in earnest, but I didn't find it as horrendous as I thought I would. I used everything I had learned in the antenatal classes and remembered how to use the gas and air correctly. My teacher had drawn a chart, and she would show the pain as a wave, signalling the point when we took the mouthpiece, making us use empty paper cups instead. We practised this every week, her coaching us to take a big breath of gas as the crescendo of pain was building and then easing off as it subsided. Thank goodness I had retained all this information and could manage to use it effectively.

Eamonn was there and supportive, but I had gone into a birthing bubble, along with Maria, my midwife, and was focusing in on the energy of the pain rather than being scared by it. Maria flagged that if I wanted an epidural, now was the time before it was too late, but the idea of sitting up felt more problematic than staying where I was. I was quite comfortable in between the contractions, at one point even falling asleep for twenty minutes. Tiredness was setting in, which was going to cause its own issues when it came to me pushing the baby out.

We hadn't found out the gender of the baby. I was tempted to because any excuse to make interior design and outfit choices, but I'm glad we didn't. It made the delivery part all the more special. Everything was going well, but then the baby got stuck. I was pushing and pushing and feeling exhausted and nothing was happening. Suddenly, there was a whirl of action, and the paediatrician came in with the ventouse machine, to help me deliver the baby. Eamonn and I went from being a couple to being a family of three and I am forever in debt to all the wonderful staff at the NHS Kingston Hospital maternity unit.

They popped the baby straight on me and said, 'It's a boy!' It was an unbelievable moment. I had secretly wanted a boy. I never said it out loud for fear I was carrying a girl, and she would know and think I was disappointed, but it was safe to share now the baby was here.

It was evening by the time baby Jack and I were moved from the birthing suite into a room of our own, just in time for *Coronation Street*. I was ravenous and the nurse said I had missed dinner, but she would see what she could find me. She returned with a mug of hot tea and a sandwich, which was synthetic white sliced bread with a thin slice of cheese in the middle, wrapped in cling film. It had that sweaty squashed look of something that had been hanging around a while, and it reminded me of picnics my mum would make us when we were little. There was also a bag of salty square crisps. Let me tell you, it was the most delicious meal I have ever had in my life!

Maybe Baby

I spent the rest of the night lying on my side, staring at Jack in the bassinette by my bed. I couldn't believe he was mine. I had a baby! A real living person who I had to keep alive. Someone I could watch and help grow and thrive, a child to adore. The pain of childbirth disappeared. I thought of the little romper suits I had packed and brought with me and the nursery I had decorated, like I was playing at dolls, while a little voice in the back of my head was saying, don't forget this is for a real baby. It wasn't make-believe. Here he was, and I was the luckiest woman in the world.

Instead of going straight home, I decided to spend a few days recuperating in a private wing of the hospital, where Maria was on hand if I needed her. She showed me how to bath Jack and helped me with breastfeeding, which I found so hard and painful. When anyone came to visit me, instead of me having to run around tidying the house, making myself look presentable and putting the kettle on, I could stay in bed, and a tea tray would be brought in for visitors. Who would ever want to leave instantly and go home with a tiny baby?! I didn't have a big support network and Eamonn had to go back to work, so I knew once I left, it was all on me.

When I talk to other mothers about this time in my life, it resonates. Most of us just wanted to stay in our pyjamas, go at the pace of our small sleeping and sometimes screaming babies and recuperate. There is nothing more stressful than knowing people are popping in to see you and needing to look like you are coping. As I tell pregnant women now, don't get dressed or put a cake out if you don't feel like it because it may discourage people from going home! There really is no need to rush around.

Back at home, Jack was unsettled. I was breastfeeding him, but it wasn't going well. Breastfeeding is such an emotive issue, and women can feel anything from incredibly disappointed to a complete failure if they have issues with it. This could be physical or emotional, but the point is what's best for baby, which means they are well fed and thriving with a happy mummy, so if this is achieved by incorporating formula or giving up breastfeeding entirely, then so be it. Sometimes you have to know when to stop and eventually I did. A friend of mine had so much milk she could have fed all the babies in the maternity unit, but that doesn't happen for everyone.

I was in love with my little boy and living one day at a time, so when I finally looked at my diary I had a bit of a shock after being in a baby bubble for a few short months. In agreeing to the next series of *Loose Women*, I stupidly hadn't thought about the timing of it all and suddenly it was imminent. I knew I wanted to go back to work, I just hadn't bargained on quite how fast that would happen. More to the point, I hadn't thought about childcare. Eamonn had gently mentioned it to me a couple of times, asking how I was feeling and what the plan might be, and all I could think was that I didn't want someone else looking after our baby.

I considered all the childcare options. Nursery timings were strict, which meant there was no wiggle room if work overran or needed me in early. I wanted something that would be flexible for my strange working hours, but I didn't want anyone to live with us because I like my own space. Besides, I was Jack's mum and wanted to be fully immersed in that role when I was at home. After much consideration, a day nanny felt like the best and safest option, and we hit gold with Victoria, who was fantastic.

The other issue was that *Loose Women* had moved to Norwich, and I had to travel there from London each week, bringing Jack and Victoria with me. I couldn't bear to leave him behind so I thought this would be the answer. My fellow Loose Woman, Kaye Adams, had also just given birth to her daughter and I recently found a photo of us at the studio, both holding our babies when they were a few months old. It transported me back to that time, when I would be in the studio and Jack would be in a hotel room with Victoria. I found it impossible to concentrate on work because he was just down the road and I wanted to get back to him. I was torn, and in the end we decided it would be better for Jack to stay at home and for me to go away for one night a week. Luckily, quite soon after, the programme moved back to London, and I breathed a huge sigh of relief.

I knew I wasn't going to be a full-time stay-at-home mum. I also knew the grass was not greener whichever side you were on, working or not. I was in a very fortunate position that I could pick and choose my jobs a little, which meant I could manage how much time I spent away from Jack and get the best of both worlds. That said, in my industry you can't stay away too long or the good stuff will begin to pass you by. Also, as a freelance presenter, I didn't get paid maternity leave so I couldn't disappear for a year and expect that TV would be there for me when I got back.

Whatever my next steps were going to be, I had my son. There will never be anything, career or life experience-wise, that comes close to him. Being a mum changed my priorities and my perspective on life.

6

Being a Working Mum
(the juggle of guilt)

Jack and I did a lot of stuff together while he was growing up. Recently, I asked him if he remembered how we would often get the train on a Sunday to Waterloo Station so he could look at other trains, all the platforms and the enormous buffers. He was obsessed with *Thomas the Tank Engine* and wanted everything associated with it, including a hat and rucksack, which he would always wear on our weekend railway excursions.

Unsurprisingly, he didn't really remember because he was so little, but I do. Sundays would loom large when Eamonn was away in Northern Ireland seeing his three older children, and I wanted to find interesting ways to keep Jack entertained. I worked all week, so the weekends were precious mummy time for me.

As parents, we may think we are creating a core memory for our children, but that's not really how it works because we don't get to choose what stays in their minds. Jack will now often ask me to tell him stories of his childhood because he thinks the ones about his 'terrible twos' tantrums are hilarious. They weren't nearly as funny twenty years ago.

He wasn't badly behaved very often, but when he was it was volcanic, in a 'swiping everything off the table' or 'pulling my hair' sort of a way. Like watching the Hulk transform from a mild-mannered chap to a raging whirlwind. I told my best mate, Sam, who is Jack's godmother, and I could tell she didn't quite believe me, only ever seeing sweet, adorable Jack. She has two boys (my godsons) – Charlie is a year older than Jack and Max a year younger – and I would call her up asking if she had experienced the same tantrums with Charlie. She said only occasionally, but they were easily dealt with. I think she thought I was exaggerating, until she came to stay one weekend.

We wanted to buy Charlie and Jack some Wellington boots because we were going somewhere very muddy and neither of them had wellies. We popped to the large Mothercare store, expecting to be in and out in a matter of minutes, except I had forgotten there was a toy section in this particular branch. So using great parenting skills and blatant bribery, we promised the boys they could choose something small if they were patient throughout the foot measuring and wellie boot fitting. Which they were. So far, so good.

We went to the section that had the 'ten pounds or under' toys and said they could pick something small. Jack ignored the brief and found a fire truck bigger than the two-and-a-half-year-old him. I began with the gentle persuasion that he wasn't allowed that, trying to distract him with a soft football instead, but that didn't work. Nothing for it but to revert to the strong parenting, which involved making Jack look at me as I firmly repeated 'no'.

'Jack, you are not having the fire truck. I told you to choose from this section here or you have nothing. This is your last chance before we go back to the car, and you go home without a toy.' He wrapped his small arms around the large truck and started to walk off defiantly with it. Sam and I looked at each other. She had a similar parenting style to me, so she was totally on board as I manhandled the truck from Jack, and we marched the boys back to the car. Poor Charlie had done nothing wrong, but Sam understood I had to stand my ground with Jack, so we left empty-handed.

I had to literally wrestle Jack into his car seat with Sam helping me, and as I tried to fasten the seat belt, Jack was grabbing handfuls of my hair. I remained calm, while he was a tornado of fury. When I got into the driver's seat, Jack started pulling his toys out of the net bag that was hanging over the back of the seat, and he threw them, with excellent aim, straight at my head all the way home. Charlie's eyes were like saucers watching this behaviour and Sam said sympathetically, 'I see what you mean now,' as a plastic whale caught me on the ear.

I told Jack, if he didn't stop throwing things at me then he would be going straight to bed when we got home, which was an annoying threat because he didn't stop and therefore I had to follow through. He was kicking and screaming as I got him out of the car and carried him upstairs, plonking him in his cot and closing the door. I sat at the top of the stairs and burst into tears. Sam came up and put her arm around me. 'Oh God, mate, I didn't know it was that bad.' Jack fell asleep and when he woke up an hour later, he was a completely different child . . . back to my sweet, lovely, smiley Jack.

Looking back, I know this was a phase that so many toddlers go through, and while I was also aware of this at the time, I knew I couldn't ignore it. I went on a parenting course, which armed me with lots of helpful advice, including ignoring tantrums and not giving them any attention. I got to test that theory a while later in Surbiton high street.

There was a lovely toy shop I would take Jack to occasionally, where he would choose another little train to add to his *Thomas the Tank Engine* collection. One Saturday morning, after a happy wander up the high street, I decided we should pop in and didn't realise my mistake until it was too late. I hadn't brought the pushchair, Jack was walking with me, and this meant he was free range and able to launch himself at the entire toy train display. He grabbed as much as he could get his hands on as I repeated, 'No, Jack, Mummy said just one, you can choose ONE. Please put the rest back.'

Of course he didn't, so I scooted him out of the shop, whereupon he lay down on the pavement screaming. I wondered how a little person could have so much rage and stubbornness and watched as families stepped over him, other children looking on in horror, my cheeks burning in embarrassment. I remembered what I had been taught at the parenting class: to ignore bad behaviour, and a telling-off is still attention. So, while staying close to make sure he was safe, I waited for him to stop. It did work eventually, but it was a very public display of tantruming and parenting and it felt like I was standing there forever as people walked past and looked on sympathetically. Or tutted loudly and judgementally. When Jack stopped, I picked him up and carried him home.

Now he is the most wonderful young man, all six foot four of him, and he loves me telling these stories, often asking me to repeat them to his girlfriend.

I remember taking Jack to *This Morning* when he was still a baby and the show announced I would be joining as a regular Friday presenter, alongside John Leslie. Then, in 2006, when Jack was four, the producers asked me if I thought Eamonn, who was over at Sky, would be interested in presenting a one-off show with me to celebrate Queen Elizabeth's eightieth birthday. We had never worked together before, and I remember being really nervous. What if we were a terrible partnership?

Luckily, the opposite was true. Eamonn is brilliant at live telly and our off-screen relationship translated well – so well, in fact, that we were offered more shows, eventually becoming the anchor presenters every Friday. I thought of Richard and Judy and how occasionally their marriage played out in real time, much to the joy of the viewers, watching them bicker or share personal details. This is not something you can fake and what you saw with us was what you got.

There have been lots of great partnerships on *This Morning* but there is a particular magic an actual couple can bring to the screen that can make it more relatable for the audience at home. It's a voyeuristic insight into someone else's marriage, which makes you feel better about your own, like the eternal argument about whose turn it is to put the kettle on or unload the dishwasher.

Being in a couple gave us a shorthand and a clear definition about who covered what. For example, if the subject was football, I sat back and Eamonn led. If it was about the TV soaps, then I would take the reins. Eamonn was a seat-of-his-pants kind of presenter, spontaneous in his work and a very good listener. I was more of a preparer and had read the book and made the notes. He knew a lot of people over years of interviews, so he could give an insight into who we were talking to. We were generous hosts, we had each other's backs, and we never battled between us for airtime.

The one big professional difference between Eamonn and me was that he was happy to continue talking about work when we got home. If something had gone wrong in the studio or we were prepping for an upcoming interview, he would be keen to talk it through while I was chopping the veg for dinner. Yet for me, home meant being in mummy mode and I wanted to help Jack with his homework and snuggle on the sofa with him. I needed a boundary between work and family life. Every hour away from Jack had to count and every hour with him was focused on being his mum.

To begin with, the job and parenting juggle worked well, and then, when Jack was still at primary school, ITV asked Eamonn and me to present over the summer holiday. My instinct was to turn it down. I wanted to spend the holiday with Jack. It was a dream gig, but not at the expense of the family. In my head I was planning six weeks of idyllic adventures involving picnics, kite flying and trips to the beach.

Eamonn said, 'As your husband and Jack's dad, I absolutely agree with you, but if I was your agent I would say you are completely crazy to turn this down. And the reality is, if we say no to this, our days on the programme are numbered.' I knew he was right. *This Morning* was the biggest show on daytime, and we were being offered it five days a week. What if the next couple they asked did the summer gig and were then given our Friday slot?

It took me a few days of stomping around and saying I didn't want to before I realised I didn't really have a choice. It sounds dramatic to say that my job hung in the balance, but I know how telly works, and I needed to consider my career. I had never really thought about the long term, but I could see that I needed to.

The most important thing was to make it work with Jack, and we did. He would often come into the studio, particularly if there was a guest on who he was interested in, and he sometimes brought a friend with him. He got to meet his favourite wrestler and pop bands, so for a while we were pretty cool parents!

Although *This Morning* was only on air from 10 a.m. to 12.30 p.m., we would have to be in by 7 a.m. for production meetings, make-up and to rehearse the occasional item. After the show there was a post-production debrief followed by a meeting about the following day's programme, and then we were away by 2 p.m. at the latest. Sometimes I would be back in time to collect Jack from school, but if not we had the nanny, and she stepped in to help out over the summer too.

To begin with, when Jack was a baby, I worried that he would think the nanny was his mum and I became anxious if I was late home, cursing every red light, but when I was reassured that wasn't the case, I made those car journeys count. I would do emails, call my agent, sort out work queries and then when I was home that was it. I was Mum.

I was brought up in a family where both parents worked. Then, when Julia and I came home for the school holidays, she would have a part-time job at the army supermarket, so all three were out of the house. They came home for lunch and my role was to set the table and get the food ready every day, and Mum would pay me to do that. I was too young for a proper summer job at that time, so this was a way to earn some cash.

This attitude instilled a work ethic in me and my hope was that Jack would benefit from seeing his parents in this light. Eamonn and I both come from working-class backgrounds and we are not ashamed of our roots. We always made it clear to Jack that he was in a privileged position with a lovely home and a private education. And yet he didn't choose to be born into this life, with two parents who worked in television, so I never wanted to bang on too much about how lucky he was. I just wanted him to be aware of the world around him, and we were careful that we didn't spoil him.

I did carry small but insistent concerns about being an older parent and how this may have impacted Jack (although it appears that it hasn't). If he wanted me to jump around on the trampoline with him then that was what I did, and God help my pelvic floor! It wouldn't have been top of my list of activities. I was hitting fifty, had been up since 5 a.m. and was absolutely knackered, but I never let him see that.

Jack was essentially an only child – even though he had three half-siblings who were lovely with him, there was a big age gap.

Being a Working Mum (the juggle of guilt)

I would be the one running up and down the stairs with him having a lightsabre duel, me dressed as a homemade Princess Leia and him as Han Solo. I didn't want his early memories of me to be that I was always at work and never had the time or energy to play when I got home.

Once he was in the garden with a few friends who had come over, and they were all doing cartwheels. He asked me if I could do one. 'Can I do a cartwheel? Of course, watch this!' I launched myself, looking like it was the easiest thing in the world, until, mid-wheel, I thought, what the hell am I doing? Spraining my wrist was what I was doing, but I didn't let him know that. I didn't want him to think of me as an old mum, even though I was at least ten years older than the other mums at school.

I know it will sound schmaltzy to say how incredibly proud of Jack I am, but I am. He has grown up into a well-rounded adult, someone I adore spending time with and who has developed an admirable moral compass. All the worrying about me being a working mother as I rushed back into the house, desperate to take Jack from the nanny, appears to have been unfounded. He has no memory of me being late because of terrible traffic or too many red lights. He was warm, fed and loved. This reminds me of being a child and moving into a house that felt like home without remembering the bad stuff about it.

I don't want to be gender-specific here, but my experience around the work/parent juggle is based on female friends and women I work with. I'm not saying it is not difficult for fathers too, but this was how I felt. When I talk to women who are about to become mothers, I say 'don't overthink it'. I wish somebody had said this to me when Jack was a baby. I once walked into the loo at work and found a young producer sobbing. She told me she was just back after maternity leave and hated leaving her baby. I gave her a big hug and told her how I knew the feeling all too well and that she mustn't beat herself up about it. My advice was to take one day at a time and not think too far ahead. The important thing was to be in the present, focused on work when she was there and on being a mum when she was at home.

It's so easy to give this advice and trickier to take. The truth is, whether we work full time, part time or are a stay-at-home parent, we will always question our decisions. I am not sure I ever fully let go of the guilt and worry that I was doing it wrong, but I am here as proof that we can muddle through, and things turn out OK. More than OK, in fact.

7

What's the Worst That Can Happen in Sequins?

I love music and I love dancing. When I am at home, my playlist is on at full volume, and I bop around my kitchen. It's such a fun, feel-good, stress-relieving thing to do, as I bust some moves and shimmy to the beat. I like to think I have rhythm. In fact, I was so convinced of this natural ability that I thought I might be quite good on BBC's flagship entertainment programme *Strictly Come Dancing*. It's one of my absolute favourite shows and I am mesmerised by how the dancers move, coupled with the sheer unbridled glamour of the ballroom. So much so that I knew if they ever asked me to take part, I would jump at the opportunity.

Over the years I was presenting on ITV's *This Morning*, we would often interview the *Strictly* judges, celebrity contestants and incredible professionals, and I always loved it when Anton Du Beke came on. He was so warm and friendly. I would tell him how keen I was to learn to dance and be on the show, and in return he would take hold of me and whisk me around the floor. It was all a bit of fun, until 2017 when my agent got a call to ask if I was interested in taking part in the fifteenth series.

You'd think I would have jumped up and down with glee and immediately bought some leg warmers, but my instinctive reaction was to say thanks so much for asking, but no, no, no. Imposter syndrome again! I used my lack of availability as an excuse in my head. I was far too busy doing my day job and live daytime telly wasn't going to present itself, now was it? I thought about Jack, now fifteen, and how little I would be at home for him. More to the point, how absolutely mortifying it would be for him to watch his fifty-seven-year-old mother being swung around on Saturday nights. While there was good reason behind these concerns, I knew with some careful planning and long days I could probably make it work. The truth was, I was scared rigid, just like those first days in the Westward studio.

It was like I had gone from flirting with *Strictly* to then rejecting them the minute they asked me on a date. As with *This Morning* and the summer holiday stint, Eamonn talked me round. He couldn't understand my sudden reticence, and he reminded me how many years I had been saying I wanted to do it.

'If you say no now,' he said, 'they might never ask you again. You might regret this decision and always wonder if you would have had the time of your life. You could be good at it!' He had a point. I thought, I am just going to have to make the logistics work and suppress the rising panic. After all, I was no stranger to these feelings of inadequacy and each time I had come through the trepidation and out the other side into something wonderful. Maybe this would happen again.

What's the Worst That Can Happen in Sequins?

In the meeting with the *Strictly* producers, they made it very clear that I couldn't choose the dancer I wanted to be paired up with – but if I could wave a magic wand then who would I point it at? Easy answer. Anton, of course. Apart from already knowing him a little and seeing how encouraging and kind he was to his celebrity partners, I didn't want someone young and hot. Sorry, Anton, if you are reading this, because you are totally divine, but the fact was I was heading towards sixty and I would not have felt comfortable grinding up against a twenty-five-year-old – which my teenage son would have to watch. Probably through his fingers.

I announced I was doing *Strictly* live on *This Morning* and knew there was no way back once the words had come out of my mouth. The next step was for all the dancers and contestants to get together for a chemistry meet, where the celebrities stood in a big circle, the music played, and the professionals boogied from one of us to the next. We danced with each of them and this way the producers could look at compatibility, chemistry and height. I thought all the dancers were fabulous and it felt like a privilege to be in this space with them, but my eyes were on the Anton prize. I could see him working his way around the circle and when he came to me, I knew I had to get my game on and pull out all my best moves. I think I may have thrown my arms around his neck at one point in what probably looked like a 'hands off he's mine' manoeuvre.

I had no idea until the night of the launch show, live on air, who I would be dancing with. Everything is so excitingly secretive about *Strictly* and we were even given code names for rehearsals and wardrobe fittings. I was in the final group to get my partner, and I was standing in front of three possibles, with Anton among them. I had watched other contestants and dancers being paired up and there was a lot of whooping and jumping into each other's arms, which was fun, but not very me. I thought to myself, don't do that, don't come over all unnecessary, just look happy with whoever you get given and react in an excited yet elegant manner. Maybe a hug but keep it low key.

They called out my name and there may have been a drum roll. I'm not sure I drew a single breath in that time, until they said I was partnered with ... dramatic pause ... 'Anton Du Beke!' My calm walk towards him suddenly turned into an ungainly run, like a cart-horse, and I launched myself at him. Except I didn't leap high enough so instead of hooking my legs around his waist, I ended up with them around his thighs, and he was hanging on to me for dear life. I think this took me more by surprise than it did him.

Inside, I was thinking, 'Ruth! What the hell are you doing?! Don't jump! You never jump. Oh, dear God, you've jumped . . .' It was too late. I had committed and then I had to pretend this was what I had planned to do. I can't watch this back now because it makes me cringe. Of course, when Anton recounts the story, he adds all sorts of embellishments including a part where he staggers backwards as I cling to him. He sometimes tells it at his theatre shows and once, when I was in the audience, he got me up on stage to replay it. He makes me howl with laughter.

What's the Worst That Can Happen in Sequins?

After I had got over the shock of my behaviour, I was absolutely thrilled. Anton is, hand on heart, one of the nicest, kindest, loveliest people I have ever worked with, which I think was crucial to have in a professional dance partner. He never once raised his voice in the rehearsal room, indeed he hardly raised an eyebrow, and I gave him much cause to. He could tell when I was tired, and I would regularly burst into tears of frustration, which he dealt with in an understanding way. And he was funny. Which was a relief, because it's an intense experience, and I was pushing myself far beyond my comfort zone while also juggling two day jobs – *Loose Women* and *This Morning* – as well as being mum to a teenager. Anton had just become a dad to his adorable twins, so he must have been exhausted too but he never showed it.

I would get up every day at 5.15 a.m. to head to the ITV studio, come off air at lunchtime, grab something to eat in the car and arrive for rehearsals at 2 p.m. We were based in the atmospheric Dance Attic in Fulham, and I felt like I was in an episode of *Fame* because it was full of young, lithe dancers in leotards arriving for auditions or warming up before rehearsals. It made me want to run outside in a tight tracksuit and roll around on the bonnets of cars like they did in the show in the 1980s. There was a tiny café downstairs, run by a lovely man who served delicious homemade food and gorgeous cakes, and we would often pop down on a break. I was fascinated by the dance world and would ask everyone what they were up to, what they were auditioning for and if they had got the job.

The last thing on my mind at this point was the live show on Saturday. My focus was entirely on learning the steps and I picked them up fairly quickly, but I discovered that I was not good at retaining the choreography. This was a minor disaster. As life skills go, it's not terribly important, but if you are signed up to dance on one of the biggest shiny-floor shows on telly with millions of viewers, it's a bit of a catastrophe.

Anton would show me a dance – say the Charleston or the samba – and I picked up the basic steps quite quickly. He would be pleased and then he would put the moves together and that was when I fell apart. I just couldn't remember if I was starting from the right or left foot. I went blank. I might do something, and he would say, 'Oh, that's good. Not what I taught you . . . but still good!' He never made me feel stupid and he could see how hard I was trying. I always say that if something fails in my career, it won't be because I didn't put the work in. I give everything I tackle my best shot.

After rehearsals, I would go home and practise in my kitchen before putting my sore feet in a bowl of iced water, as advised by Anton. When I went to bed at night, I was still doing the strange dance counting in my head. Very quickly, I realised that me dancing around my kitchen to James Brown was not going to cut it here. Just because I could get up at a wedding and confidently hit the dance floor did not mean I could step out at *Strictly*, having mastered the unending amount of technical detail, and wow the judges.

I secretly hoped I would be the oldest female contestant because I could use that as an excuse, but Debbie McGee was there and pipped me to the post. Plus, she was amazing and could get her leg up by her ear.

'Oh great,' I said to Anton, 'so I am not the oldest and I am certainly not the youngest. I'm not a pop star, actress or comedian.'

'So, what does that tell you?' he asked.

'I don't know,' I replied morosely.

'It tells you to be yourself,' he said, 'just be yourself, that's all you can be, and we will have a lot of fun.' This was to be a seminal piece of advice for me, but first I had to come at it the hard way.

Soon that dreaded time was upon us, the first live show. Everything backstage was amazing, I loved it. The production crew, hair and make-up and wardrobe, they all make it the incredible experience it is and the often-repeated cliché of us feeling like part of a family is absolutely true. It was a new insight for me into the world of glamour and entertainment, and I lapped it up, with dancers whooshing in and out of the dressing rooms, sequins sparkling and a sticky veil of hairspray hanging in the air. When they danced, I was transfixed by them and I thought these magical creatures might stay separate from the rest of us, but they were so welcoming, and we became one big gang.

The costume department blew my mind. They created the most incredible outfits and would sew us into our dresses (and have to patiently cut me out again when I needed a wee, which was often!). I am not a cleavage girl, I like a sleeve, and I don't like things slashed to the thigh, and they respected that, but still managed to create dresses that made me look and feel sexy. Most importantly, I had to be able to move in them. The make-up team were my first port of call on Saturdays, and they also kept me calm before the results show when I was convinced I would be in the bottom two and therefore going out. Their unruffled attitude and brilliance meant we kept in touch, and I still work with some of them to this day.

I hadn't realised how different it would be, from dancing with Anton in our tiny studio in Fulham to turning up at a huge studio full of people and cameras. I had been in a little bubble all week and that instantly burst when I faced what was next.

There is so much to organise and do before the live show that it's easy to forget what is coming until the Friday of studio rehearsals. This is when the crew do the camera run, sort out the rigging and give each couple two practice run-throughs in the space. There was no audience but there were a lot of people mooching about and I froze. The choreographer, Jason Gilkison, was brilliant and tried to put me at my ease, telling me to ignore everyone around me who were getting on with their jobs, explaining what was going on. 'Just do your dance,' he concluded. If only it was that simple.

The music started and it was like my entire memory had been wiped. I could not remember a single step of the waltz. I kept stumbling, going in the wrong direction and treading on Anton's feet. He didn't make any jokes, he was speechless for the first time, and I thought I was going to cry in front of the crew. Jason scooted over and told me not to worry, that the first rehearsal was often terrible, which was why we got another chance to go through it. Anton agreed and they both gave me big smiles of encouragement. Considering Jason had to think about every dance couple, I will never forget the kindness he showed in a moment that was undoubtedly stressful for him too. Second time around was better. It wasn't brilliant, but it was enough for everyone to feel relief, me included.

To cheer me up, Anton told me about a celebrity contestant he had one year who whispered in his ear just before their first dance began that she couldn't feel her legs. Poor woman, I thought, and was glad that this wouldn't happen to me – I got nervous doing my day job, but I never suffered from stage fright. Anton sent me home saying, 'Tomorrow you will be fabulous, in your beautiful dress, lovely long hair and sparkly make-up. Absolutely nothing to worry about. Now go and get a good night's sleep.'

I barely slept a wink. I had got myself into this situation and now it was the worst part. Be careful what you wish for because you might just get it. The day went by in a whirl of action and nerves, helped by the rest of the lovely contestants, who were all in the same boat. Although the live show didn't go out until around 7 p.m. it was a very long day for all concerned, going through make-up, wardrobe and full dress rehearsals.

We waited behind the scenes for the theme music to begin, the signal we were live to the nation (how many millions I did not want to know), swiftly followed by the introductions as each couple came to the top of the stairs and glided down. Anton had tight hold of me, he could feel me shaking and he told me how gorgeous I looked, reminding me to smile as the camera focused on us. I did a stupid little wave, which I would never normally do (what was wrong with me?!), and then we walked down the stairs, me praying I wouldn't fall. I really did not feel like myself.

Our dance was scheduled towards the end of the show, so we stood up in the balcony, watching each couple and cheering them on. Every contestant looked amazing to me. They really were all outstanding and, as time passed, my nerves got worse and worse, and I had a deep sense of dread in the pit of my stomach. I eventually turned to Anton.

'I can't remember the dance, the steps, it's all gone out of my head,' I said. He looked at me, and he could see I was panicking.

'Come on.' He grabbed my arm, pulling me away from the action. 'You don't need to see any more of this.'

We went downstairs to the little tea- and coffee-making station and Anton suggested we have a cuppa and walk through the steps.

'Ruth,' – he was very calm – 'you do know the dance. And even if you don't, I do and I will just guide you around the floor so there is nothing to worry about.' I thought, he's right. Thank God, of course he knows it, and he will be right by my side.

When it was our turn, Tess Daly announced us and a spotlight shone brightly on our fixed grins before they rolled the VT (a pre-recorded piece) of me crashing about in training and I could hear my voice saying, 'I am so excited to be on Strictly, it's my dream!' In that surreal moment, it felt like an utter nightmare. It was at this point my brain seemed to detach from my body. As I walked down the stairs to get on the dance floor, I was aware of just how many people were in the studio. I live and breathe live television so that wasn't a problem, but I had never performed in front of a big audience before and I swear I could see the whites of their eyes. Everyone was staring at me. I could sense them all willing me on and wanting me to do well, which almost made it worse because I couldn't bear the idea of letting them down.

Our dance began just in front of the orchestra (who gave me a little supportive wave). There were a few steps up to a little stage where a chaise longue was positioned for me to sit on demurely, waiting for my suitor – Anton – to appear. Then I was supposed to get up and walk towards him down the steps, where he would take my hand, whirl me around and whoosh, off we would go. Here started the longest seconds of my life. I couldn't move and I felt dizzy. I had no saliva in my mouth, so my smile was more of a grimace with my lips stuck to my teeth. My heart was beating so loudly I could hear it in my ears, and I was convinced the audience would be able to hear it too. And I thought, I am going to faint. Right here, on *Strictly*. A live show. Nobody has ever done that before, it would be a first. Maybe they'll cut the cameras or focus on the judges? Everything about the experience, from how I looked to what I was doing, was so alien to me.

I had spotted Eamonn and Jack in the front row and, unbeknown to me, at that moment Eamonn turned to Jack and said, 'I think she's in trouble.' He could tell from my wide-eyed stare. The music began and Anton danced over to me and held out his hand, which I didn't take. I didn't move. History was repeating itself for him because I couldn't seem to make my legs work, it was as if my feet were blocks of concrete. I just looked at him like I had no idea what I was doing there, as if someone had just plonked me down on the chaise and told me to stay still. He came up the stairs, took my hand and pulled me up, making it look like this was the choreography we had always planned.

I remember him taking me in hold and then it became an out-of-body experience, as if I was watching myself from the corner of the room and in my place was a rag doll, being carried around by Anton. I think he did just lift me off my feet at certain points. All I remember is the advice he had given me in rehearsal that 'whatever happens, remember to smile because if you look uncomfortable the audience will feel uncomfortable watching you'. I tried to show the composure I was far from feeling and grinned like a Cheshire cat!

The finale of the dance was three big twirls – something I was good at because Anton had taught me those early on – while fireworks went off behind us, and then we returned to the chaise, where we had started. At this point I came back into my body, relieved that I hadn't thrown up or collapsed, but with no memory of what had just happened. We stood in front of the judges, and I smiled and nodded a lot because I couldn't catch everything they were saying. It was like listening to a radio being tuned so I would get snatches of their conversation and then it would disappear again, and I was just watching their mouths move. The next thing I knew, we were back upstairs with Claudia Winkleman, and I thought – or maybe said out loud – 'Oh my God, I have just danced on *Strictly!*' Then I definitely said, 'I was terrible!', to which Anton said, 'Nonsense, you were stupendous' in his hugely supportive way, hugging me close and defending me against judge Craig Revel Horwood's low score.

What's the Worst That Can Happen in Sequins?

If that was my first time and I was convinced I was going to die of nerves, how could I do this every week? Anton was going to hate me. I was going to hate me. What I realised in hindsight was that I had suffered a panic attack, not something I'd ever experienced before. The only time I could remember a feeling of sheer terror that came close to it was in the early days of my screen career when I was pushed on to cover for Roger, the continuity announcer. It also reminded me of a number of actors I have interviewed over the years who talked about stage fright, with one saying she had to throw up in a bin every night before she went on stage. I now appreciated what they were talking about. As a presenter, I often have the buzz of adrenaline, but this is usually a powerful feeling that keeps me on my toes and helps me be good at my job. It's a positive energy, unlike the awful disconnect that overwhelmed me in the first live *Strictly*.

Anton was unperturbed. He congratulated me on getting through the debut performance, said I looked lovely and that from now on it would be much easier. He always made me feel like I had done a fantastic job even when I knew I hadn't, and he was there to calm my nerves and boost my confidence.

We moved on to the second week and while I still felt ill during the live show, it was a little better than before. We soon got into a pattern, but I struggled with the choreography. I was so embarrassed that I couldn't seem to keep it in my head and so frustrated it would make me cry. Anton named those days Teary Tuesdays and Weepy Wednesdays, the low points of learning a new routine. We started every Monday with a new dance, say the tango, and spent all week on it, before the live show on Saturday. By the following Monday I had to forget all about the tango because we were on to the foxtrot. It was incredibly stressful at times, but Anton always defused these situations with a gag or words of kindness. If he hadn't, I'm not sure I would have been able to continue.

In week five, we were in dress rehearsal dancing the samba and Anton was in the most ridiculously brilliant outfit of an orange and pink shirt with massive frills on the sleeves and pink sparkly trousers. He was bouncing around in front of me, giving his encouraging smile, and I had an epiphany. I finally saw the joy of it.

'Ruth,' I said to myself, 'look, you're not a dancer. You're not very good but just let yourself go because look at him. He's smiling and laughing because this is a FUN dance. And so what if you get the steps wrong? You're here now so just let yourself go.' It was a privilege to be there, and I didn't want to waste another second on the negatives. I just had to be myself.

From that moment, the abject fear evaporated. Yes, I was still nervous every Saturday and yes, I never completely knew my dance, but I found the compassion for myself and the love for what I was doing. Maybe if I had had more hours available for training things would have been different, maybe not. Perhaps I am one of those people who just can't keep the choreography in my head. I will never know because I won't get the opportunity again, but I was so grateful to have had it in the first place. Let me go back for another shot at it! Surely I would be better second time around!

What's the Worst That Can Happen in Sequins?

I look back now and can't believe I lasted for nine weeks, although I wish we could have stayed in one more week and got to Blackpool. I think the viewers kept us in because they liked our partnership rather than admiring my footwork. The highest score I got from the judges was 6 for my tango, four 6s in fact, and I was thrilled. Craig Revel Horwood had given me a 2 at one point in the series and when I saw him in the bar after the show, I jokingly said, 'Two? Really?! Do you know how hard I have worked?' He gave me a big hug. 'Darling, you know I love you,' he replied, 'but it was dreadful.' And I had to agree with him. I adore Craig for his humour and honesty.

I found the hardest dance was the rumba because I had to be sexy and there was a bit of gyrating. It was Movie Night week and we were given the James Bond theme, dancing to *Diamonds Are Forever*. At the beginning of the dance, I had to run my hands seductively over my body and then walk down a set of stairs. This worked well in rehearsal, but in the live show there was billowing dry ice, which I was not expecting. I had to try to look sultry, while desperately searching for the stairs with my feet. Bruno Tonioli, one of the judges, called me an ice maiden – 'Dahling,' he said, 'your hips were frozen stiff, they need thawing out!' It was funny and I didn't take it to heart – after all, it's an entertainment show.

The funniest moment for us as a couple was the paso doble, which seems to have become an iconic moment in the show's history. At the end of the dance, Anton wanted a big finish with me lying across his knee, but in the live show he lost his balance and toppled backwards. There was a split second where I had to make a decision about how I would react. I decided to lean into the comedy of it all, so I climbed on top of him. There is a brilliant picture of my bum in the air and Anton's feet sticking out from the bottom of my skirt. The place was in uproar! The camera panned to Eamonn and Jack, who were laughing together. They knew me so well and saw I was trying to manage what could have been a really awkward moment by making it funny. I think this, more than anything else, showed how far I had come on my *Strictly* journey.

As for my lovely boy Jack, it can't be easy having two parents on TV, let alone discovering that one of them was going to be dancing on live telly every Saturday. He was a teenager who could be mortified by a lot less so I was worried about how me being on *Strictly* would affect him, particularly the amount of time it would take up. I did speak to him about it before I signed up and he was happy for me to do it. I needn't have been concerned. He came every single week. Every time the camera panned to him, he looked so proud, and it made me cry. That was the best feeling for me, that I had his support – he was really upset for me when I was finally voted out.

It's nice to write about *Strictly* here because I don't get to talk about it that often. As each series comes around and new celebrities put on their dance shoes, my time fades into the background. Occasionally, someone will even say, 'You should do *Strictly*.' And I say, 'I did!' It was everything I hoped it would be and more. I give Anton much of the credit because he transformed my time on the show from an experience I wasn't sure I could get through to the most joyous challenge I have ever taken on. He was also as truly himself off-screen as he is on it. What you see is what you get with Anton and that can be a rare thing in our industry. He was my teacher, protector and biggest cheerleader and we are still friends to this day.

The realisation that I could have allowed fear and nervousness to ruin my time on the show could have come sooner, but thank goodness it came at all. I channelled my dear old dad and Anton's wise words about having fun, and repeated to myself, what's the worst thing that can happen here? Well, the worst would be dropping dead, which wasn't likely unless I was terribly unlucky. OK, so yes, I might faint, but the crew would just cut to a VT or fill the time in some way. So what was I worried about? Making a fool of myself? Not being very good? Well, I wasn't very good because I wasn't a dancer. Nobody was expecting me to look like a professional and I knew we weren't going to win. In which case, what did I have to lose? And this attitude released me from the shackles of my own agony.

Let's be frank. I work in entertainment. I am not saving lives here. I am not performing heart surgery. Or going down a mine. Yes, my fear was disproportionate to the situation I was in but that didn't make it any less frightening.

I could have said no to *Strictly*, maybe I would have done if Eamonn hadn't given me the gentle nudge I needed, and I would have missed one of the most amazing times of my life, which I will cherish forever. It is like being part of the best club in the world. I found it hard to watch the following year because I was filled with envy. I didn't want to see Anton dancing with anyone else, it was like he was cheating on me! Despite my childish jealousy, I was thrilled for him and his new partner, actress Emma Barton, who was brilliant, and I happily cheered them on to the final.

Looking back on that experience, I remember Anton's advice to just be myself, which can sometimes be the hardest thing to do. I was concerned about who I was on *Strictly* in a way that I had never been before. What you see of me on screen as a presenter is who I am in real life and when someone says this about me, it is a huge compliment. But being your true self when you are far out of your comfort zone is difficult to achieve and the show was such a learning curve for me. It taught me to believe in myself in unfamiliar situations and not be scared to look stupid.

It's OK to be afraid of things, it's a human reaction to challenging times, but it's how you deal with it that counts. If fear is holding you back and stops you doing what you want to do, then it could be time to take stock. Maybe just asking ourselves 'what's the worst that can happen?' might be enough to help us face the fear and do it anyway! I gained such a huge sense of pride in myself, and I thank Anton, Eamonn and Jack for all their encouragement because I doubt I would have done it without them – and what a regret that would be.

8

Thanks for the Memories

Had he still been alive, my dad would have been tickled pink to see me on *Strictly*, but at least I had my lovely mum and sister there, cheering me on as always. I know how lucky I was to have the family I did. I was always close to my parents and loved going back to visit once I had left home. It felt like going to see old friends, the sort who also cooked your favourite food (shepherd's pie followed by vanilla ice cream with a dollop of clotted cream on top), included you in their daily crossword chat and whose company you never tired of. When I lived in Plymouth, just over the estuary from them, I would visit and still stay the night, and they would also come over to see me on Dad's motorbike. Like sixty-something versions of Hell's Angels.

Then things went a bit pear-shaped. My lovely dad was diagnosed with Alzheimer's when he was in his early seventies. We had suspected it for a couple of years and even before then we'd been aware of small, odd behaviours, which we had put down to ageing or low mood. By this point, I was living in Surrey and working for ITV, and my sister, Julia, was in Sussex, so we weren't seeing our parents on a weekly basis.

On one occasion, I went home for Mum's birthday, and we took a day trip from the south coast of the county to the north, to visit a National Trust garden she had been longing to go to. On the way there, Dad took the main roads and then we returned home across the moors. I was in the passenger seat next to Dad and Mum was in the back. We drove past a farmer leaning over a five-bar gate and so Dad waved, and the chap waved back. It was the sort of thing my gregarious life-loving Dad often did.

'That's funny,' Dad said after we had driven past, 'because he waved to us on the way up and he's still there.'

'No, Dad,' I said, 'we didn't come this way this morning.'

'What are you talking about, Ruthiee? Don't be ridiculous. This was the route we took earlier too.' Dad was beginning to get cross. We often butted heads because we were similar characters, and I loved a good old debate with him where neither of us would back down. Sometimes I would say stuff just to wind him up, but this was not one of those times. Mum, ever the peacemaker, shushed us both, and I should have let it go, but I didn't.

'No, we didn't, Dad.' I was insistent. Surely he couldn't have forgotten which way he had driven? It was only a few hours ago.

At home I got the map out, still determined to show him I was right.

'Dad, here was this morning's journey' – I traced my finger along the roads we had taken – 'and you must remember because we passed here, and here on the main road. Then on the way home, we drove across the moor. You see, you couldn't possibly have seen that farmer before because we were nowhere near his farm.'

He refused to believe me and then I said it. The thing that still haunts me now.

'Jesus, Dad, are you going mad?!'

It would be another five years before he was properly diagnosed, and I look back at that incident and several like it and part of me is furious with myself. I handled it so badly and should not have let my irritation show. What did it matter, was I just trying to win the point? And yet I am empathetic to my naivety, particularly now I know what was to come.

I lost count of the number of warning signs we had. Mum saying Dad had lost his camera, for example. Dad never lost anything. He lived by the motto 'a place for everything and everything in its place'. He was incredibly organised and if you stood still long enough, he would label you, which is where I've obviously got it from. If anything was out of place he would be infuriated, and there was a regular refrain of 'who's had the bloody Sellotape?'. His camera was always in a cupboard on a shelf marked 'cameras'. They hunted high and low and eventually found it in the fridge. This would be a tiny bit funny if Dad was a chaotic person, but he wasn't so this was a worry. Particularly as he was furious with whoever had put the camera in the fridge because he said he knew for a fact that it hadn't been him.

Now, I always say to people who suspect a loved one has Alzheimer's that they know them better than any doctor, and if that person is behaving out of character then this is a big indicator. My dad was incredibly sociable and loved a spontaneous road trip, taking Mum to a garden centre or the cinema, but he suddenly stopped wanting to go anywhere. At first, we three women of the family wondered if he might be depressed, not knowing that dementia is often mistaken for depression.

When we realised he was forgetting things, I fought hard against this. I thought I was helping him by trying to jog his memory, pleading with him to remember old family stories as I gave him more and more pieces of the puzzle or showed him photographs. He just looked at me blankly. I wish I could go back and tell myself to stop, that this wasn't helping him and nothing was going to bring those memories back. It would just end in frustration and distress for us both. Sometimes we would argue. What a waste of precious time together that was.

The trigger for suspecting Dad had dementia was a strange car he bought. He was a great driver, was never happier than when he was on the road and enjoyed being behind the wheel of a nice motor, so this weird hybrid of van meets car was very out of character for him. I could tell by Mum's voice over the phone that she was concerned, but she was fiercely loyal to him and didn't want to draw attention to it.

The next time I went to see them, the first thing that struck me was the car. It was so unlike anything Dad would choose, yet he seemed happy enough with it. As a military man, he was a stickler for cleanliness, but this vehicle had escaped his high standards, and he didn't appear to notice how knackered and grubby it was.

'This is a bit unusual for you, Dad,' I said, gingerly getting into the passenger seat.

'Oh, I think it's quite nice,' he replied.

'Really?' I said. 'I don't think it is.'

He drove to the supermarket, a place they had been going to every week for many years. We bought what we needed, and on the way home we got to the big roundabout and he stopped. I was mid-flow, chatting about something or other, and I looked at him. He was just staring straight ahead as the cars backed up behind him.

'Dad? Are you OK?'

He frowned. 'Now, which way is it?'

'Er, straight over.' I couldn't believe he didn't know, he drove this route all the time.

'Oh yes, course it is,' and he sped off without looking. On the main road he drove at snail's pace, but once we got on to the country lanes, he was too fast, scraping the side of the car against the hedgerows.

When we got home to my parents' little bungalow, I was amazed that we were both still intact and I went into the back bedroom to phone my sister immediately.

'Julia, something's not right here. Dad's not right,' I said. And that was the beginning of the downward slide.

The GP referred us to a dementia specialist, who came to the house to do the tests with Dad. By this point, he didn't question it because his brain was not functioning in the way it used to, so he just thought it was a regular check-up with a new doctor. The specialist asked him to count backwards from one hundred and Dad was proud that he had done it so easily. Maths had always been his strong suit. However, he didn't know what month it was. Or what day. The specialist was kind but to the point. Yes, it was Alzheimer's and no, there was nothing we could do about it. No medication, no intervention.

Dad could do crosswords quite late into his Alzheimer's. He became obsessed with them, starting years earlier with the puzzle in the *Daily Mail*. He got to the stage where he didn't really read the paper anymore, he just waited for it to drop through his letterbox, sometimes pacing the hall until it arrived, and then he would settle down with the crossword. This became one of the important routines of his day.

It took Mum a while to get her head around Dad's illness. She had put a lot of it down to him being distracted, tired or getting older, and she didn't recognise it as anything else – or had chosen not to. Once he had the diagnosis, we encouraged her to tell her friends and neighbours. It was important for the small village community to know as they would all want to be there to support them both, particularly as Julia and I were many miles away. Mum pushed against this for a while and then a couple of things happened. One day she nipped out to get a few bits and left Dad with a sandwich, a cup of tea and his crossword. He was perfectly happy to be left for an hour. When she returned, she saw he had been through an entire box of matches, lighting them one by one and watching them burn out.

The second warning followed swiftly. Dad was no longer allowed to drive and he was incensed. He couldn't believe it, so I told him it was the law: when you got to seventy, they took your licence away. That seemed easier for him to digest than the truth.

Once, the car was in the local garage having some work done and Mum came home to find it parked outside the house.

She assumed the mechanic had dropped it back, which she thought was kind of him but unusual. It turned out Dad had gone to pick it up and had driven it back, with no licence. The thoughts of what could have happened on that short, hair-raising journey do not bear contemplating. Mum realised that she now had to hide the car keys. These are things you learn. That highlighted to us the need for everyone to know about Dad's dementia because had the mechanic had any idea, I'm sure he would not have let Dad drive off. It was a constant learning process for us all.

Much of the time, Julia and I would discover what had happened after the event. Mum said there was no point worrying us and 'after all', she often repeated, 'what could you do?' I was down one weekend and had coffee with Mum and some of her friends. When Mum went to the loo, one of the women revealed how worried she was about her, particularly now my dad was getting up in the middle of the night and falling over. Or flushing his pyjama bottoms down the loo and flooding the bathroom. This was all news to me, and I raised it with Mum on the way home, but her response was still, 'Ruth, what could you do? We are fine.'

Around this time, I was presenting *This Morning* and there was a phone-in about guilt. A woman came on, sounding very upset, and explained how guilty she felt because her husband had Alzheimer's and he had been away in respite care for a week. He was due to come home that day and she didn't want him back. She said she was struggling to look after him but felt so guilty that she was dreading him coming home. For the first time in a long time, she had been able to sleep at night. And then she broke down in tears.

Listening to this viewer be so honest and emotional unlocked something in me. I had not spoken publicly about my dad's diagnosis, but here I was, empathising with her. I said how much I understood and explained what my parents were going through. I was in tears, and so was the caller.

Afterwards, a lovely woman called Maria from the Alzheimer's Society got in touch. She had seen me talking about my dad and she asked if my mum needed any support. It was like hearing from an angel. We spoke at length and she put me in touch with the Plymouth branch of the Alzheimer's Society. They ran a dementia café, and they invited Mum and Dad along. This was a game-changer for Mum because she got to talk to other carers and get helpful advice, finding out about handy hacks and gadgets, like a mat with an alarm that goes off when someone gets out of bed and stands on it. It gave her more of a toolkit to help her deal with Dad and emotional support from people going through the same thing.

It also encouraged her to be more open with others about Dad's diagnosis. She started telling people and the local community were lovely, stopping to chat to Dad when he took his daily walk to the shop. He often forgot what he was supposed to buy so she would write a little note and tuck it in his pocket, and when he got to the shop they could ask him what Joan wanted. When he forgot that he had a note, they reminded him. Once, he fell over and somebody picked him up and brought him home. Mum tried to give him as much independence as possible until it was clear it was too much for her and was making her ill.

One night, Dad fell coming back from the loo, and Mum couldn't get him back into bed, so she made him a cup of tea, covered him with a blanket and sat next to him. She didn't want to bother anyone at 2 a.m. so she waited until it was light and then went to the neighbour. She's very stoic, my mum. When she told me, I asked her why she hadn't called an ambulance or woken up the neighbour (who wouldn't have minded), and she said she didn't like to make a fuss. 'We are fine,' she repeated, but I was unconvinced.

Julia and I looked into respite care, which Mum was dead against. We introduced it in the form of Dad being a day visitor every week to give Mum a breather. Dad railed against going but he enjoyed it when he was there, and we were always encouraging about what the place offered. Home life was getting harder and Dad would regularly lock Mum out of the house when she went into the garden. Also, he had always been such a smart, clean, beautifully smelling and closely shaven army man, and this changed. He didn't see why he needed a shower every day or to change a shirt with an egg stain down the front.

Julia and I knew, long before Mum did, that Dad wouldn't be able to stay at home. We were worried about how ill it could make her and also the level of danger that they were both facing. I had a conversation with one of the health visitors who had popped round when I was down at Mum and Dad's. She said perhaps it was time for Dennis to go into full-time care. I replied that hell would freeze over before my mum would admit she couldn't cope anymore, so we needed to move things forward in a careful way, engineering it behind the scenes. Dad went in for a week's respite, and the home said that, as if by magic, a full-time place had become available, and they thought he and Mum would benefit from it.

Mum was devastated and called Julia and me to discuss it. We told her what she didn't want to hear. 'Mum, it's time, this is making you unwell and Dad needs to be somewhere safe,' we reassured her. We couldn't force her, but we hoped she could see this was just as beneficial for Dad as it was for her. He was incontinent, often falling over, and would decide to take baths that she couldn't lift him out of. I will never forget someone at the care home saying to Mum, 'It's OK, Joan, you can go back to just being his wife now.' I found that so emotional.

Mum reluctantly agreed on the proviso that if he hated it then we could bring him home. She went in every day to see him.

I once did a campaign for the Alzheimer's Society around Christmas because they said they get a lot of calls in January, after families have been together over the festive period and noticed a loved one behaving strangely. I remember that with Dad. I always made him and Mum a Christmas stocking each when they came to stay. When I went into their bedroom on Christmas morning, it was clear that Dad didn't know what to do with it. He just stared blankly at the stocking, not understanding that he had to open it and take the presents out. This was the same man who loved Christmas and always did stockings for me and my sister. Suddenly, it had all been wiped from his memory.

Jack was two when Dad became ill. Before he went into the care home, Mum and Dad would come up and stay. One morning, Jack was sitting on the kitchen floor building his toy bricks and knocking them down again with much hilarity. My lovely dad, who in another life would have sat on the floor to play alongside him, shouted at him for being naughty. I scooped Jack up and took him into another room and Mum intervened with Dad. It was heartbreaking. Dad would have hated knowing that was what he had become; he would have been the first person to take Jack sailing and fishing. Jack never knew the man I did and when he was about seven and saw photos of his army grandad zooming over the brow of a hill on his motorbike, he couldn't comprehend this was the same man.

Dad stopped recognising us. Me first, then my sister and finally Mum. It was awful. I became the nice lady who turned up with chocolates and cake, which he was always happy about. He never asked who I was, it was just a slow disintegration, before I realised he didn't know me.

After much persuading, Mum agreed to move to a bungalow near Julia in Sussex and we moved Dad to a care home down the road from there. It meant Julia and I could visit more easily and also be able to take Mum out and spend time with her. I am so glad we did because we had the loveliest couple of years with her before everything fell apart.

When Dad died in 2012, I was devastated. He had stopped eating, and the care home warned us it would be a matter of days rather than weeks. I had just been to see him, and I had come back to take Jack and his friends on a half-term trip to

Cirque du Soleil at the Royal Albert Hall in London, they were all very excited. I spoke to Julia, and she was there with Mum. We all knew Dad wasn't great, but she reassured me there was nothing I could do. She told me to take Jack for his treat and then I could return the following day. So that's what I did, except the following morning, at 6 o'clock, Julia called me and as soon as I saw her name flash up, I knew. 'Daddy's gone,' she said.

When I arrived, Mum and Julia were there, and I said I wanted to see him. I took his hand, and it was a shock that he was so cold. I was wailing and hugging him while my sister rubbed my back. In another part of my brain, I was shocked by how upset I was. Dad had been ill for a long time, he had no quality of life, he would have hated to know this was how it ended for him, and I had prayed he would be released. Now he was, and I couldn't stop crying. I became the little girl, and he the gentle giant of my childhood. The man I adored, my fantastic, fun dad. Now I could mourn the person he used to be.

There was also a sense of relief, and my focus became my mum. She had lost her lover, best friend and life partner. The man she met at a dance and fell in love with.

Dad's funeral had a touch of the military send-off. We had an army padre, his military cap sat on his coffin and his favourite jazz music played as he left. We were asked if we wanted to speak and I said I didn't think I could. Julia and my Uncle Arthur, who is an emotional man, agreed with me, so the padre said we could write what we wanted to say and if, on the day, we felt able to read it out then we could, otherwise he would. When we reached that moment, he looked at me first, the television presenter, and I shook my head, I was in bits. Then he looked at my quiet, shy sister and she stood up, walked to the pulpit and read our eulogy beautifully. I couldn't believe she had done it.

Afterwards, holding her hand, I told her how proud I was of her, and she said she hadn't wanted anyone else to read our words about Daddy. I thought that was amazing. At the wake, surrounded by photos of Dad before Alzheimer's took him from us, we celebrated his life, a good and interesting one.

We never told Dad he had Alzheimer's. I am not sure if that was the right thing to do. Maybe it depends at what stage your loved one is diagnosed and how you feel that person will deal with the news. By a cruel twist of fate, I got to use all the lessons I had learned with Dad because Mum started to become rather forgetful. Julia and I put it down to the stress of Dad's death, but we knew the signs by this point.

This time around I didn't try to fight it or push Mum to remember things, I knew better and was well versed in what was to come. On the odd occasion when I would be trying to explain something to her, she would look at me sternly and say, 'Ruth! I am not five.' I know I must have sounded patronising and I had to be careful of the tone I was using. Julia and I went with Mum to the dementia test.

I was doing *Strictly* at the time, and Julia and Mum had come to see me in the show. We were backstage afterwards at the bar and we were chatting when Mum just blurted out, 'Oh by the way, apparently I have got Alzheimer's.' She said it in such a breezy way, and I knew then that it already had her in its grip because she seemed so unbothered and had already changed the subject. This wasn't very Mum. Julia and I locked eyes over her head and without speaking we communicated the same thing. Here we bloody well go again.

When we moved Mum from her bungalow in Plymouth to a smaller bungalow in Sussex, I was the one who had to be strict about what she could take with her. Ironic for a woman who has moved so many times in her life, but she had amassed a lot once settled, including more kitchen equipment, garden stuff and terracotta pots than I knew what to do with. The fish kettle could go. When was she ever going to cook a whole salmon again?

Mum's bungalow in Sussex was tiny, but it had a lovely garden, and we put in a new kitchen and bathroom, so she was very happy there. Julia was always around, keeping an eye on Mum without her even knowing it: checking the fridge, reminding her about appointments, making sure she took her medication, the good cop to my bad cop. I felt guilty that I didn't live closer – I was working and Jack was still at home – but I visited as often as I could and shared the load in different ways.

And then came something even more awful and shocking: Julia's death, something I have written about in a later chapter. In terms of my mum's condition, I wasn't aware of the Alzheimer's being so much of a problem because I think Julia had done much more for Mum than any of us realised and it helped mask the bigger issues around dementia. Now there was no buffer.

Without Julia, it made sense for Mum to move closer to me. I found a lovely care home literally around the corner from me, somewhere that would be able to accommodate her developing illness. She was so good about it. It was an incredibly hard time.

She had lost her daughter, and I was mourning my sister, and here we were going through all her stuff again because she was downsizing to a bedroom, small sitting room and kitchenette. Now, without my beloved Julia, I had to be bad cop AND good cop. I remember it being a sunny spring day and I had brought stickers to put on all her things. A red sticker for the pieces that were absolutely going with her, yellow for stuff she wanted to think about. I had to persuade her to use more yellow than red.

I had her new bedroom painted the same colour as the one in the bungalow and I gradually moved things over, put pictures on the wall, bought a smaller sofa, arranged flowers in a vase and plumped the cushions. I was doing what I had watched her do over fifty years before as we moved from place to place and she made each one a home. I wanted her to walk into familiar surroundings as she had wanted me to do as a child, and the emotion and full-circle nature of this was not lost on me.

I visit Mum regularly and bring her flowers and chocolate, which she loves, but she never remembers they are from me. When I arrive, she is usually in the communal sitting room, among all these elderly people who were once pilots, barristers and teachers. Money and status don't protect us from dementia. In Dad's home there was a woman who swore like a navvy and her daughter apologised to us. She said her mother had never sworn, hated it in fact, and she wouldn't allow her children to swear either. Maybe she's making up for lost time, I thought. In many ways, it seems so much harder for families to watch their loved ones being so changed by this awful illness than it is to be the one suffering from it.

When I go into the care home, I wave to Mum, and she always waves back, then I see her turning to whoever's there and telling them I am her daughter. For a moment, it's as if nothing has changed, until she asks me how I knew she was there and what a lovely surprise to see me. I have stopped reminding her that she lives there and that I see her every week, because she just looks confused. I check her room is clean, change the flowers and make sure she has everything she needs. Her world has become very small and it's my job to make sure it runs smoothly for her.

If I'm not taking Mum out somewhere or bringing her home with me, then I bring my dog, Maggie, which is very cute because they adore each other. Recently, I have felt Mum disappearing into the past. She still knows who I am, but she often asks why Dad is late home. The first time it happened it was like a dagger in my heart, and I had to stop myself from crying. Now I play along with it, saying he is on duty, so she stops worrying about him.

I think she may have regressed as far back as her childhood because she talks a lot now about her mum – my grandmother – and how worried she will be because she doesn't know where my mum is. Mum once said she was surprised that my grandmother hadn't visited her and fear made me say, 'Granny is dead, Mum.' And then I turned it into a joke, saying if she was still alive, she would be about 130! 'You are ninety-three, Mum.' Silly me, she said then, but next time she brought it up she said I was lying because Granny had been writing to her. 'How can she be dead if she writes to me every week?' Mum said sniffily.

So that is where we are now in this awful decline, and I haven't made the same mistake again. I learned from seeing Dad go through it.

The first time she mentioned Julia, she said she was surprised Julia hadn't joined us for the music event at the home because she would have loved it. I held my breath. I thought I was going to burst into tears. How could I tell Mum all over again that her daughter was dead? I just couldn't – why make her relive that trauma? My instant reaction was to protect her from the awful reality, so I was quiet for a moment and then I said airily, 'Oh, Julia is gardening today because the weather is so lovely. She has to make the most of it.' Mum nodded in agreement and tapped her toe along to the music. As her Alzheimer's has progressed, my role with Mum has swapped from being her child to being her protector.

Mum won't remember the biscuit she has just eaten, the dental appointment she has just attended or the conversation she has just had. It falls out of her head a moment later. If I try to remind her it causes confusion and anxiety, so I quickly move on, finding ways to distract her. Sadly, this is not my first rodeo and this time around I am much better at it.

In December, I drive her around the neighbourhood so she can see everyone's Christmas lights and then we end up at my house. Last year when we pulled up, she looked at the house and said, 'Ha, you don't live here. It's not possible for you to live in a house like this!' And I said I did and took her inside. Every time she comes over now it is as if for the first time, but then she remembers little things and she recognises Jack in this context too.

Feeling Fabulous

When she fell and fractured her pelvis at Christmas 2024, she was rushed to hospital. Jack was with me, and we went to visit her. She couldn't understand why she wasn't able to get out of bed, repeatedly being reminded that she'd had a fall, like new information all over again. Jack sat on one side of her bed, and I sat on the other, and she looked from me to him and then said, with an eyebrow raised, 'So where did you two meet?'

I am asking her more about her childhood now. Even if I already know the stories, I love hearing them again and she is happy and safe living in the past. The thing I find most difficult is leaving her because she doesn't think she is at home. Before, she understood why she was there but now she doesn't, and so as I get up to go she thinks she's coming with me. It was so tough for a while, but now we have a routine where one of the carers comes over to take her to the dinner table and I say I have to take the dog out for a walk. I tell her I'll see her later and leave the room without looking back. I hate it, but I think it's the kindest way to do it for us both. She won't understand any explanations, and it is likely to create a scene. Before I go, I spy on her through the hatch into the dining room and I see her chatting to someone sitting next to her.

I don't dwell on whether I will get Alzheimer's as both my parents did. I don't want to know if it is in my future – unless they discover a cure for it – and I don't want to spend my days waiting to see if it's going to get me. Occasionally, my mind will go completely blank, and I forget someone's name or where I have left my keys, but that could just be a busy brain. Maybe I am tired? What about the menopause? Or just getting older?

We all get these moments. I don't spiral down a hole of fear, because I have a big life to live for as long as I can.

I miss my family so much. Our little unit of four. My hilarious dad, my kind mum, my loving sister. All the special occasions we celebrated, the annual theatre trip and afternoon tea for my mum and sister's birthdays. The traditional Christmas shopping day with my dad, when we would end up in the pub in the evening surrounded by bags. Time makes everything feel easier, but it never goes away. With Mum, I have an acceptance that I never reached with Dad. I was angry. Where had my fun dad gone, the one who used to turn the music up loud and dance around the kitchen with me?

It's hard losing the person they were. I was in denial with Dad and wanted to battle the disease, but I am much kinder to myself now and just enjoy being with Mum, sitting next to her, doing the crossword together, as much as she is able. I try to live in the absolute moment with her because that and her past are all she has. I hold on to the memories of who she was, the creative homemaker, always in the garden or on her allotment, cooking, sewing all our clothes and decorating the house seasonally with her fabulous Easter, Halloween and Christmas tables. I have inherited her beautiful decorations, which I put out at those times of the year, and I enjoy continuing the traditions she started. I know she would have been chuffed about that.

I am an ambassador for the Alzheimer's Society, after their early show of support, and for the last fifteen years I have been part of their annual Memory Walk. It's a lovely thing to do for various reasons. Not only does it feel like a tribute to my parents, but it's also a privilege and an inspiration to meet so many other people who have been affected. Yes, it's emotional, but it is also very uplifting. Whoever you walk with you start chatting to, and they are very open; everyone has a story and a person they are walking for. I met a woman who had been diagnosed with early onset dementia, and she was just fifty-seven. She told me she was in shock and had to give up her job because her brain just couldn't cope.

Mum and Julia used to do the walks with me and Jack has been coming since he was small. I remember one around Plymouth Argyle football stadium, and Painshill Park, down the road from me in Surrey, used to host one too. I always give a speech before the start of the walk. Interestingly, considering I'm an over-prepper, I never write my speech, I just try to speak from my heart. Talking to people I meet and listening to their experiences is all the support I need. I talk about my dad, which brings a lump to my throat, and now, when I mention Mum, she always gets a cheer from the crowd.

On those walks – and whenever the subject of Alzheimer's comes up – I say the same thing. There is no manual or blueprint for living with or dealing with someone with the illness. The important thing is to try not to feel guilty about whatever decision you make. It's easier said than done. When Mum was in the early stages, she would still come to my house for Sunday lunch, and I would occasionally post something on Instagram of us dancing in the kitchen or chopping veg. Somebody commented that if I loved my mum so much then why had I put her in a home. I was raging. I try not to take any comments personally, but this one was a bright-red rag to an angry bull, and I responded saying they had no idea of my mum's needs and what it would take for her to live with me. A full-time carer, for a start, someone with medical knowledge. Mum rattling around an empty house while I am out at work. No activities with fellow residents. No music events. No stimulation. I know she is better, happier and safer where she is, but my guilt makes me question it. So, when I tell people not to feel guilty, I am really telling myself too.

I also remind myself how lucky I am. Mum is not in pain, she is happy, she still knows who I am, she has a great sense of humour and she's living in her memories. The staff always say how lovely she is, and I can see how they are the same with her. She once told them she had just got back from Singapore and I explained that it wasn't a complete fabrication because she did live there, it was just a very long time ago, but that is her reality now. She is time travelling.

There is more awareness of dementia today but still not enough, and certainly not enough funding for desperately needed research. The Alzheimer's Society has been such a brilliant resource for our family and supported Mum in the early days, telling her about claiming for care allowances and helping with paperwork. I recommend them to anyone who needs a listening ear and a guiding hand.

This is one of the heavier, more painful sections of my story, but I do feel it's an important one. Of course it is personal, because Alzheimer's has been a big part of the last twenty years of my life. Also, and I know this is a big fat cliché, if this can help someone else who is dealing with a newly diagnosed loved one and wonders what the hell is going on, I see you. I understand. I hope sharing my experience is useful. And I dedicate this chapter first to my darling dad, who I hope is scrambling around on motorbikes wherever he is, and second to my wonderful mum. Just the other day she mentioned how much she loved the apple cake her mum used to make and it wasn't a story I had heard before. It was lovely and I hope I get to hear many more of her memories.

9

When Endings Become Beginnings (in three parts)

Part One: The dreaded empty nest

When Jack left for university, I did not expect to be quite as upset as I was. After all, he was a normal teenager who spent a lot of time with his friends or in his room, so he didn't hang out that much with us. When other parents said how they hated the silence in the house once their children had left, I didn't notice that as much as his lack of presence. He just wasn't around. The place felt different, empty, as if everything was paused and waiting for his return. His coat and bag weren't dumped in the hall, there was no wet towel left on the bathroom floor and his trainers weren't a trip hazard at the bottom of the stairs. After years of nagging him to tidy up his clutter, I was bereft without it and him.

In the weeks before he left, I was in full organisational mode, just as I had been when I planned out his nursery eighteen years earlier, forgetting that I was bringing a real, live baby back to it. Now, I was busy ordering bed linen, labelling everything and buying kitchen equipment without thinking about what that actually meant. I even bought him a nice tissue box cover! In my head, I was playing house. In reality, Jack was leaving home.

Jack went along with my planning, including the cushion buying even though he wasn't bothered about them (further proved when I found them stuffed under his bed when I went to visit). He is an empathetic, intuitive person and I think he could see that me sorting stuff out for him was a deflection. He didn't get impatient or cross with me about it and I buried my head in the sand by choosing a duvet cover. Yes, he was grateful for the help, but also yes, I should have stepped back and left him to it a bit more.

It's important to share how we feel at these junctions in life. While it's a thrilling, liberating point in our children's lives, it is also scary for them, and it can feel like such a shift in the family dynamic and a loss for us parents. I know some don't feel the same conflict of emotions and I understand that too, but for me it was a body blow. We get over it, but not before a little wallowing in the misery. Sometimes, empty nest is referred to as a 'living loss', which may sound rather dramatic to some, but it made sense to me. Why should I be embarrassed to admit that I cried for a week when Jack left home?

I was so proud of him and happy that he was off to study broadcast journalism. It turns out he is a chip off two old blocks, but we had not encouraged this pathway, he had chosen it. I wanted my wonderful boy to fly and begin his brilliant adult life. My work here was done, except those of us with older kids know that it never really is and they come back a lot during uni years (the summer holidays are long!).

When Endings Become Beginnings (in three parts)

Taking him up to university in Salford felt more like a jolly road trip, not a drop-off, and I was focused on settling him in his room, helping him make his bed and unpack his clothes. It was so exciting for him, and I didn't want to ruin it by blubbing everywhere, but I could feel the emotion welling up between us all. Eamonn and I said goodbye, got into the car and both promptly burst into tears. As we drove off, I looked up to the seventh floor where his room was and I could see a hand at the window waving goodbye.

Back at home, I went into Jack's room and sobbed. I buried my face in his pillow and felt the terrible ache of missing him. In those first few days, I was very wobbly, and I kept his bedroom door shut, figuring that I could just pretend he was still in there. I tricked my mind into imagining he was watching telly, playing a computer game or had popped out to see his mates.

After a week, I felt better, but I hadn't spoken to Jack since the day we dropped him off. I didn't want to be the annoying mother who was constantly checking up on him, so I had let him be. I knew he would call me when he was ready. Then I found out Eamonn had spoken to him. Jack had rung to talk about the football, and this was a dagger to my maternal heart. I needed to know if he was OK, happy, settled, eating properly? 'We only really talked about the football match. He's fine, Ruth,' Eamonn said. What sort of a word is fine?!

My friend Sam, the one who witnessed Jack's terrible tantrum the day we went to buy wellies, has a theory about boys going to university. She thinks they are more likely to cut the apron strings immediately because they don't want to be mothered anymore, so they disengage for a while. Her son did the same. It doesn't last, but it feels a little brutal at the time.

This made a lot of sense to me, and I thought about how I should deal with my communication with Jack. I had a backlog of questions that mainly consisted of whether he had been eating green vegetables, had he worked out how to use the washing machine, did he remember to use the fabric softener I had left him, how was freshers' week and had he made any nice friends? I would likely have asked all of these and more without drawing breath. I could see how this might be annoying for him. No wonder he called Eamonn to chat about the football. It was a safe conversation without any fear of his dad asking if he'd put the washing machine on the right setting.

When Jack did ring me, I stopped myself from asking any of those 'mum' questions. Keep nonchalant, I reminded myself, let him chat, don't scare him off by asking if he has eaten any fruit that day. It was so lovely to speak to him, but I was careful not to gush and after a while I said I had to go. I didn't want him to regret having called me or be put off the next time for fear I would be naggy or nosy. We agreed to catch up again at the weekend and then I came off the phone and the tears flowed. He called me more regularly after that.

A while ago, Jack and I were reminiscing about his university days and the terrible timing with the pandemic and lockdown when he was still a fresher. He casually slipped into the conversation that he had had Covid when he was there. I couldn't believe he hadn't told me at the time!

When Endings Become Beginnings (in three parts)

'Because, Mum, you would have jumped in the car and raced up with chicken soup and tissues. You wouldn't have been allowed in, and I was absolutely fine. I took a couple of paracetamols and went to bed for a day.' Probably just as well I didn't know.

At least I didn't have to worry about Jack and food. He really liked cooking when he was little and loved helping me in the kitchen, pulling up a little stool to stand next to me. And he did food tech at school, bringing delicious dishes back that he had made, so I was pretty sure he could fend for himself.

Once he was settled into uni life, he cooked more and I loved the messages that started, 'Mum, when you make your Bolognese, do you put the onions in first?' He sent me photos of what he was cooking, often using family recipes, which made me rather proud. When he was home in the uni holidays, I couldn't wait to cook for him, starting the day with a big breakfast while he sat at the kitchen island. Even now, I am never happier than when Jack is home for the weekend and I am wielding a frying pan while he sits and chats about his life and job in Manchester. I think he loves it too.

When Jack came back at the end of the first term, he was different, older somehow. He seemed much more mature, even though he was still a teenager. He was telling me about his friends and for the first time in his life, I didn't know them. They weren't the mates I had known since they were small, who came round and lounged on our sofa or disappeared up to Jack's bedroom. He hadn't known anyone going to the same university, but he made new friends quickly, partly helped by joining the hockey club. Through each stage of university, be it in halls or then a shared house, he was happy and fulfilled and it was all I could have wanted for him. It didn't mean I didn't miss him though.

Saying goodbye to him after each break when he returned to uni was incredibly hard. No sooner had he settled back in at home than he was gone again. It didn't seem to get any easier. I cried a lot, but for a shorter amount each time. Always as he drove off, and even now, he beeps his horn and blows me a kiss out of the window, and it makes my heart break a little. The tears are a combination of missing him already and the fear around him getting back to Manchester safely. He always texts me to let me know he has arrived. It's something I did with my mum too. I knew she would be worrying but wouldn't want to make a fuss. That doesn't change, no matter how old your children are.

Yet in an ending comes a beginning. And here also comes a generalisation. Women can be very good at putting everybody else first. Our parents, our children, our partner, our boss, our friends, our neighbours – and before we know it, we are at the back of a very long and demanding queue. As we get older, I think we see this and feel it more. We are tired, frustrated, resentful and ready to burst forth!

In the days of a young family, work and general business we don't have time to wee let alone think, but things change. This is one of the positives of the empty nest, it gives us room to spread out. Without the school run, without having to cook every night, without the arguments over homework, screen time and curfews, our lives expand. We need to ask ourselves, what

When Endings Become Beginnings (in three parts)

do WE want to do with the next stage in our lives – and then we must grab it with both hands!

Part Two: The ebb and flow of a career

A change in your career can bring a similar sense of loss to that of the empty nest. It might prove to be the beginning of an exciting new era, but it's still the end of something familiar and happy. I loved *This Morning*. As cheesy as it sounds, we really were one big family. When our resident agony aunt, Denise Robertson, died, we were all devastated. She was such an amazing woman, an integral part of the show, and epitomised the camaraderie among the team.

I had the best time on the programme, from 1999 to 2022, and it continued longer than I could ever have hoped for, so I am eternally grateful. Nothing lasts forever, particularly not in show business, and when it ended I was incredibly sad and cried on my last day, but I carry the most amazing memories of my time and the brilliant crew I worked with.

We never knew exactly what we were going to get on the show because of its response to current affairs and the magazine angle it took, so it was always interesting, busy and fun. The cookery section was one of my favourites and there were chefs who taught me dishes that I continue to cook. I loved the fashion segment too, which is now reflected in my work at QVC (a shopping channel). And gardening, which I knew a little about, and it always reminded me of my grandmother, my mum and my sister, generations of great plantswomen. Then if there was something big happening, a breaking news situation say, we had to scoop it up and respond in real time, which got the adrenaline pumping!

I still miss *This Morning* and I will forever be one of its cheerleaders and alumni, but the time I have gained since leaving has been channelled in other happy directions, like QVC, *Loose Women* and writing this book. So many new paths to travel and silver linings to be thankful for.

A while ago, I went to my *Loose Women* friend Janet Street-Porter's brilliant one-woman show, which was classic Janet in a dry-witted, irreverent way as she shared anecdotes from her life. It was impressive that she remembered so much, but she has kept a diary since her teens, and I really wish I had thought to do the same. I could have noted all the good times and the amazing people I met. There is so much I forget or have a hazy memory of, particularly in my career.

The entertainment industry, like many others, has been struggling recently and I have colleagues and friends who have lost their jobs. I reassure them that something else always comes along. I don't want to sound flippant or uncaring because I feel the opposite, but I speak as someone who has lost her job several times in her life and somehow managed to get another one. I am still here. And while a lack of work can feel like the end of the world right now and you wonder if you will ever work again, you will. It may not be your dream job and sometimes it has to be something that will pay the bills, rather than the work you have trained for and love, but the trick is not to give up hope and to continue to strive.

When Endings Become Beginnings (in three parts)

Part Three: Heartbreak

OK, so let's tackle the elephant in the room. The breakdown of my marriage, which has been the focus of almost every press story about me for the last couple of years. At one of the hardest points in my life when I wanted to run away and hide in a cave, I was faced with regular news pieces about what was perceived to be happening in my relationship. Kind friends said, 'Ruth, don't worry about it. You know what they always say about the press, it's tomorrow's fish and chip paper!' But it isn't, not anymore, it's carved into the internet forever, ready to be regurgitated in the next article and the next. You only have to do a quick google of me and several inaccurate stories pop up.

I am not complaining. It comes with the job, and I know the score. After all, I worked in a news environment back in the day, under pressure to get the next exclusive. I understand how it works. I have also seen it in action in a tabloid newsroom, walking into an office full of people wearing headphones and watching TV screens. *Loose Women* was on one of them, which was a surprise to me, and the journalist told me they were watching so they could pick up any choice comments for instant online fodder and possibly the next day's paper.

As a country, we have a huge appetite for gossip and my personal situation appeared to tick several juicy boxes, but the reality was quite different. Now look, I know some will want the full story in gory detail while others don't give two hoots. The truth is, I am not going to delve publicly into something when it involves other people. What I can talk a little about is how the separation affected me emotionally because I know those who are going through this may find it helpful. It's also important to me that I can pull out the positives from an awful experience and encourage others to do the same.

The biggest emotion that threatened to swallow me up in the early days was sadness. When you have been with somebody for a long time – twenty-six years in our case – and had imagined what your future would look like, there is a sense of deep loss to know that this has changed. I expected Eamonn and me to be together forever and knowing this was not going to happen was incredibly hard to come to terms with. Suddenly, life was different, with no clue what the months and years ahead would look like.

I was devastated in the beginning. We had gone from being a couple, traversing the usual ups and downs of a marriage, to an abrupt end. This was how it felt to me and it was a huge shock.

There can be a lot of doom-mongering at the beginning, and there certainly was for me. So many concerns whirled around my head. What if I couldn't cope on my own? What if I were lonely? What if I would never meet anyone else again? What if I lost my job? What if I got ill and there was nobody to care for me? I was already without my sister and my dad, and my mum was lost to her memories. It was a scary time, following on the back of a huge amount of loss. In talking to others going through break-ups, I knew I wasn't alone in my fears, and this reassured me. It helped me realise that worrying about things before they happen or that are unlikely to happen is a waste of energy at exactly the time you need to be firing on all cylinders. Yes, I

When Endings Become Beginnings (in three parts)

needed to grieve for what was lost and could have been – but I had to look at the life I still had and how I could make it whatever I wanted.

In short, I gave myself a stiff talking to and not just once, but many times. By worrying I couldn't cope, what I was really saying was I couldn't cope without a man and that was ridiculous. 'Pull yourself together, Ruth!' I sternly instructed myself. One night, in the early days of being alone, I was watching TV and all the lights went out. There was a moment of confusion and then I thought, it's bound to be the circuit. I knew where the circuit board was and I knew what to do and I realised that I had always dealt with this, I didn't need a husband to gallop in on his white charger.

Eamonn and I would laugh about the fact that when we first met, I had a toolbox and he didn't. He said if something small went wrong in his flat – a broken door handle or a rickety shelf, for example – he would call someone to mend it.

'Why?' I asked. 'When it's just a screw needed. Where's your toolbox?' He looked nonplussed.

'Oh, hang on, I think I have one in the car,' he said. He came back with the socket set.

'That's not a toolbox!' I laughed. 'I'll bring mine next time I come over.' My dad was the most practical man ever and had given me everything I needed, including a screwdriver and hammer, and then taught me how to change a plug.

DIY is not gender-specific. It is not a boy's job to hang pictures or replace a washer in a tap. We should all know how to deal with small maintenance jobs around the house. It helps that I am one of those naturally practical people. I am not helpless, and I would do well to remember that. I also think it's worth making the point that we should all have a toolbox and an understanding of how to use a drill. The sense of liberation I get when I mend something far outweighs many of my bigger achievements!

Now, I know what I am about to say is another of my big fat clichés, but it is also the truth. Time is a great healer. It absolutely is. No amount of rushing will get us to safe ground; we have to wade through the swamp first. One day, almost without realising, we will feel a little better, a little brighter. We will find we can laugh easily again and remembering something poignant will make us smile rather than cry.

While we are stuck in the swamp, we can find therapy and support in all sorts of places, whether this is with a trained counsellor, a bunch of girlfriends over a couple of bottles of wine on a Friday night or a dog sleeping at your feet. All these things work, or at least they did for me.

I didn't want to go to a therapist, but a friend of mine who had been dealing with a similar experience said she wouldn't have got through her divorce without a bit of professional help. I didn't think I needed it. I didn't need a counsellor to tell me what I already knew. Put simply, I was incredibly sad that my marriage was over, and I needed to come to terms with it, so I resisted the idea for a while, thinking I'd get through it just fine, thank you. My friend kept trying to persuade me, saying I could do one Zoom session and if it didn't feel comfortable or I didn't gel with the therapist then I could stop. 'If it's not for you, then

When Endings Become Beginnings (in three parts)

I will shut up,' she said. Curiosity and my determination to get better meant that eventually she did manage to persuade me. One session, I thought, then I can say I gave it a shot. I knew it wouldn't be for me.

I loved the first session, and I loved the therapist. Nobody was more surprised than me! So I kept going back even though I was sure I wouldn't need it for long. For the first three Zoom appointments, the therapist only saw the top of my head because I was crying so much. She said to me, 'Ruth, this is grief. This is trauma and you are in shock. Let it all out.' It was as if I had been waiting for permission to be upset and acknowledge the monumental fallout from the marriage break-up.

I found there was a big difference talking to someone impartial rather than speaking to my loyal, wonderful girlfriends, who are always on my side. It didn't feel fair to keep offloading on them either. Therapy gave me a more measured view of the situation and the tools I needed to be able to deal with it. I was in no rush to give it up, but there came a time when I knew I didn't need a session every week, so we did every fortnight and then we went down to one a month. This was another reason I liked my therapist so much – because she understood what I needed and when I was ready to try standing on my own two feet.

I am not happy my marriage is over, but I have accepted it. I think this has been the biggest turning point for me because fighting against the inevitable is exhausting and pointless. For anyone going through similar, I would urge you to find your peace with it because this is about creating a new but just as worthwhile life as a single, independent person. It doesn't mean you aren't hurting, but you have a choice. You can fall apart and not get out of bed in the morning, or you can get up, have a little weep and keep going.

There was often a moment on waking when I would forget what had happened before reality came rushing in. My time to cry was in the shower in the morning, when I would sob loudly and snottily. Once I was out, it was time to pull myself together and say firmly, 'That's enough now, Ruth.' Nobody had died. This was another new day. Get in the car. Off you go to work. Come back from work. Have a little cry in an empty house. Cuddle the dog. Cook dinner. Watch the soaps on TV. That's how I dealt with it, and I don't know of another way because I have no desire to take three months off and go trekking in Thailand to find myself, eat, pray, love style!

Instead, I didn't make any major plans. I took it slow and steady. Running away from things only means that you have to face them when you get back. The pain, anguish and frustration are all still there, just like the bins that need to go out and the laundry that has to be done. Best to hunker down and find a way through; and now I am out the other side, maybe I will go to Thailand for a holiday and visit my best friend. I can see a new, exciting chapter of my life stretching out ahead.

I can still be caught out by the emotion of the last couple of years. I'm not sure you can live with someone for that long and not be. It can floor me, and when this happens I take a few deep breaths and a moment to gather myself before getting on with the day, my job and family stuff. Some people have said how

When Endings Become Beginnings (in three parts)

tough it must have been to go through this while I had to put on a smiley face on telly, but it would be no different if I worked in a bank or a supermarket, for example. It's my job and there are many times I have been grateful for the distraction. Thank God for work!

Empty nests, job loss and divorce all figure highly on the list of most stressful life experiences, along with the illness and death of someone close. I have had all of these, and I am here to tell the tale. I am here to say that while it is awful, devastating and can feel impossible to survive, you can, and you will. Trust me on this.

10

She Looks Good . . . For Her Age

I know I shouldn't take any notice of what people say about me, particularly when they are complete strangers, but in these times of the internet and social media, it's not always easy to avoid. The other day, for example, someone called me Wrinkly Ruth. Yep. The context was even worse because it was linked to a story about my marriage break-up and they said, 'Good on you Eamonn, for getting rid of wrinkly Ruth.'

I know a troll when I read one and I rarely look at the comments. I have been in the public eye for a long time, and this sort of heckling comes with the territory, so I am used to it. And yet this insult infiltrated its way through my thick skin. 'The truth is,' I said to myself, 'I am quite wrinkly.' And just like that, I went from feeling fabulous to falling into a tearful slump about ageing.

I realised they had hit a nerve, which was why I was upset. If they had called me Stupid Ruth, I would have taken no notice because I know I am not stupid, but they threw something at me that I couldn't easily bat away.

The ageing process is highlighting parts of myself that I have never thought about before. I know I should just give myself a break and I never notice these things with others, but I am self-conscious about my neck, particularly if the camera gets too close. It's all I can see on screen.

I work in an industry where a lot of people choose surgery. There is nothing quite as exposing as television (and the way it can add ten pounds and show every single wrinkle and the turkey neck) or the dreaded red carpet at high-profile events. I haven't had Botox or fillers. I am often tempted and never say never, but taking such invasive action doesn't sit comfortably with me. No shade on others who have 'tweakments' and plastic surgery; each of us needs to feel empowered to do what we want to our own bodies and faces. I am more interested in the motivation behind it. Are we doing it for ourselves, are we doing it for men, or are we trying to keep up with other women? Perhaps all three. Although I would be tempted to say it's more likely to be for other women. That is where we may fear judgement and feel the need to be in the tribe, which can mean wearing the right clothes and looking a certain way.

I am sixty-six. This is how I look, people! When we say that someone 'looks good . . . (pause) . . . for their age', what is that age supposed to look like? My mum's generation had a sort of uniform of elasticated slacks, comfy shoes and short hair that they adopted at retirement, but thankfully times have changed, and our wardrobe can be a reflection of who we are whatever our age, not who we feel we should be. Let's not ask ourselves if this dress/skirt/top is appropriate, let's ask whether we like it and if we feel good in it.

We may be better at not defining people by their appearance, but weight, looks and age are still matters for public and media debate and for our internal monologue. We can tell people to #bekind and #loveyourbody but this is #bullshit because most of us don't love our bodies. Of course, it is brilliant if you do and you are the sort of person who genuinely doesn't care about your size, shape and ageing. Good for you! I salute you and I am also hugely envious because I don't feel like that.

In fact, I'm a bit sick of being told to love my body. I will decide if I do or I don't and at this age, I don't love it. There, I've said it. This isn't just about growing older; I have never been #bodyconfident. Even in my youth, I wasn't a skimpy dresser who was relaxed about displaying lots of cleavage and I never wore really short skirts. My idea of a hellish invitation – then and now – would be to a pool party where I might be expected to lounge around in a bikini. Like those Ibiza raves where everyone is bouncing about in thongs the width of dental floss or lazing around in *Love Island* with a #beachreadybody. That sort of situation would have me running for the hills. No thank you very much.

Some years ago, I was asked if I wanted to take part in a body-positive campaign, which would mean having a photo taken of me in my bra and pants. I said no for a couple of reasons. First, my son, Jack, was a teenager at the time, and I don't think he would have appreciated seeing his mum plastered on huge billboards in her underwear. Or how he would feel going into school knowing all his mates had seen it too. Secondly, the premise of being aware of our bodies is tied into being completely in control of them and making our own decisions. It was my prerogative to say no. That's body positivity for me, not to feel the pressure to embrace the bits of myself I am not fond of. I know how empowering that is for some and I champion them, but I do not want to strip off, and I hope this attitude can also be respected.

There is such a pressure on women to look good whatever their age, and looking good basically means to look slim, fresh-faced and youthful. Personal grooming, from dyeing hair and false nails to fillers and face lifts, is a continually growing and evolving industry, targeting women far younger than is healthy. Sometimes I would pick Jack up from school and all the girls coming through the gate looked so glamorous. I didn't have my nails done until I was in my forties and the first proper pedicure I had in a salon was when I was pregnant. I am so glad I didn't grow up against the backdrop of expectation of beauty perfection and social media judgement, particularly as I had my own insecurities to deal with.

I have never thought of myself as a natural beauty – I need to put in some work to help me feel more confident. Whether that is to blow-dry my hair and pop in heated rollers or put on mascara, it takes maintenance and effort. I can't roll out of bed and out of the house. This has nothing to do with the industry I'm in and the job I do. I have always felt like this; it is part of who I am.

If I am at an event, Ruth from the telly kicks in and I make sure I have done my hair and face and chosen an appropriate outfit, often clothes from my own collection at QVC. There's something of the fairy tale about my job and needing to look as people expect me to. I find it inspiring when I see other women looking great, so I know it matters.

She Looks Good ... For Her Age

I was once invited to the Brits, many years ago. Only once. I'm not sure why they asked me or why I accepted, but the thought of hitting the red carpet at this sort of achingly cool event sent me into a tailspin. It seemed fashionable at big music events to look like you hadn't made an effort, but that wasn't very me. I knew my usual glitzy frock choice wouldn't cut it, so I opted for a leather blazer and then spent the entire night thinking I looked like someone trying too hard.

In contrast, I have been to the National Television Awards over the years many times, an event I enjoy and feel comfortable at, but the red-carpet angst remains the same. I always plan to lose some weight in the run-up and then I forget about it and suddenly it's the week before and I have to tear around in a panic trying to find something to wear. This is what happens to me, and to many of the women I know, before any big event like a wedding or a party.

Getting ready is a big old palaver, even when I have a helping hand (several) for something like the NTAs. The event begins at 6 p.m. so I have to start primping at lunchtime. The glam squad pitch up to my house to do my hair and make-up, for which I am eternally grateful; they get me into my dress, sparkling jewellery, a pair of heels, and then I am in the car and on my way. I have to sit bolt upright in the back because I often have my hair up so I can't lean on the headrest in case it messes with the perfectly coiffured look. The dress is usually uncomfortable because the bodice is tight so I can hardly breathe. And then I hope to God I don't need a wee before I get there. I have been known to stop at a roadside garage and swish out in a long dress, desperate to find the loo and feeling ridiculous.

Once I get out of the car at the event I can feel the anxiety rise, because all I can see is a bank of photographers and flash, flash, flash on one side and then lots of people on the other side with camera phones. There is a moment when I check myself. Hold in your stomach, Ruth. Where is my bag? I hope my hair looks OK. Don't fall over! I hate this! Why do I put myself through this?! And then I'm off, posing for the photographers, chatting to reporters on the red carpet, being on my guard for any sneaky questions, stopping to talk to the crowd and have selfies taken. I would love to see the result of those hurried phone pictures because they are probably of my ear or up my nose.

Now, here is what we must all remember, whether we are going to a party, a wedding or wafting down a red carpet: looks are deceiving. There is usually somebody extremely glamorous in front of me who appears to have no fear about the red carpet and glides along it looking amazing while the photographers fall over themselves to get the best shot. I wonder, if I were to stop those women (and men, but let's face it, mainly women) and ask them how they are really feeling, how many would say they are racked with nerves, haven't eaten for two days, are sure that everyone can see the big spot they have tried to cover up and feel their dress is too short/exposing/tight/boring/flamboyant? I would put a large bet on the fact that many of them feel like me.

We shouldn't compare ourselves to other people and think they have found their fabulous because they are slimmer, taller, prettier, wear lovely shoes and are always smiling. I know I am guilty of this and social media doesn't help as it gives a constant window into other people's lives. Many of the high-profile people we follow have had a lot of help from hair, make-up and wardrobe stylists, and I speak as one who knows. As tempting as it is to turn up for work and go straight into the studio, I'm not sure you would want to see me in my curlers, no make-up and an old sweatshirt with a coffee stain down the front!

The first time I ever walked the red carpet, I was completely clueless. I had chosen a peacock-green/blue satin cocktail dress, which I loved, yet when I saw the pictures the following day, I thought I looked terrible. I was so upset. The camera flashes had caught the satin in such a way it made me appear as if I was six months pregnant, and I looked startled, like a rabbit in the headlights, my nerves clear to see. I had no idea how to stand for the cameras and I have learned the hard way, by seeing awful photos of myself looking like a sack of spuds. I watched how other women did it: one hand on the hip, lean on the other hip, shove that hip out and put one leg in front of the other. It looks ridiculous in real life, but somehow works on camera.

I remember worrying I was fat. I look back and think, I wish I was that fat now! What the hell was I worried about?

This is absolutely not a complaint about red-carpet anxiety. I love my job, and this is a privileged part of it. I never forget how lucky I am to be invited to these events. My point is not what I am doing, it is my attitude to myself while I am doing it. I think I can give myself an incredibly hard time before an event and imagine I am the only person who feels vulnerable on the red carpet. My worries really stem from how I look and, more importantly, how that will be perceived. Will I be in the press the following day for being one of the worst dressed? Did I get it right or wrong? Will the picture haunt me on the internet forever more?!

The media aren't quite as cruel as they used to be. I remember one headline, attached to a photo of me with a protruding tummy, stating that I had 'embraced my curves', but what I think they were implying was that I looked fat. I was called Curvy Ruth, which I guess is better than Wrinkly Ruth.

Then there was my gorgeous red evening dress that was rather low cut, which was unusual for me, and it was quite expensive, so I wore it to several different events. This resulted in an article that basically said *Gosh, Ruth really likes this dress, doesn't she!* as they listed the number of times I had been seen out in it. What felt like a sly dig actually backfired because I am very proud of re-wearing my clothes from an economical and sustainable perspective, and I was not about to be shamed for it.

Of course, to quote Oscar Wilde, the only thing worse than being talked about is not being talked about, and the morning after a big event there are likely to be a lot of high-profile people and their stylists checking to see if they made it into the press. I confess that this used to be me, slightly disappointed the following day if I hadn't been featured somewhere after running the gauntlet of the red carpet. I would think, well, what was the point of all that then? Sometimes the pictures surface months later in weekly magazines, where they choose a photo to try to match the story of whether I am 'broken-hearted', 'moving on with my life', 'dishevelled', 'smug' or 'fuming'. I find it amusing, which is just as well because I can't do anything about it.

She Looks Good . . . For Her Age

Men do get an easier deal, and they don't tend to start getting ready six hours before an event. I hate to say it but there we are, and I wish there was an equivalent female version of the tuxedo. A suit or a black dress that we were allowed to wear on repeat and look the same as the woman next to us. Maybe just change the tie or jazz it up with some jewellery.

How we look is still a big part of what defines women. Forget the reason why we may be at an event, everyone just wants to know where the frock came from. And do you look good? Do you look hot? Do you look young? Do you look thin? Even better if the evening ends with a shot of someone falling drunk into a taxi with someone inappropriate! I must make a note to try that some time. Joking! Or am I . . .

I don't tend to go to many industry events. I have never been a big networker with a grand master plan. I don't make strategic connections or show my face in useful places. I have made some great friends in telly, and they are real relationships with people whose company I enjoy. I am firmly in the JOMO (joy of missing out) camp, without any twinges of FOMO (fear of missing out).

All of that said, I am about to contradict myself because I know I need to make a little more effort and say 'yes' to the lovely invitations that really appeal. I need to be careful not to just head to my sofa every evening, as happy as that makes me. I do need to push myself out of my cosy little nest once in a while now I am single.

As for being off-duty, I have got better at not giving a damn about how I look when I'm going about my everyday life. Of course, some may expect me to look a certain way because of what they see on TV or in the magazines. Sometimes people's disappointment is palpable if they bump into me in the frozen aisle at Sainsbury's and I am in joggers and trainers, with my hair in a ponytail.

'Oh gosh, it's you,' they say with an expression I know only too well after all these years, 'you look so . . . different.' And I guess what they sometimes mean by 'different' is: not glamorous with professionally groomed hair and make-up and wearing a nice frock. Early on, I decided not to let this worry me because it would look stranger to go to the supermarket looking like I was going to a wedding.

I have always been on the back foot with how I'm supposed to look and felt I was bigger than most of the women in my peer group on TV. I'm quite tall and the slimmest I've been is probably a size 10 but more like a size 12. I have never been thin, and I am fine with that, but the menopause has made it much harder for me to manage my weight.

Growing up, weight was never an issue for me. We didn't have a lot of money so treats were sparse. There was a sweet tin that lived on a high shelf and every Saturday we were allowed to choose a few sweets, which were carefully counted out. Crisps were a rare offering, and fizzy drinks poured out sparingly at the weekends. Mum loved Dandelion and Burdock, which I thought was disgusting, so we had nuclear-green limeade or a neon orangeade instead, which was delivered by the Pop Man. During term time, the boarding school canteen provided meat and two veg type meals, with no snacks, so I wasn't an overweight child and I don't remember any of my school friends talking about diets or having food issues.

This might be one of the reasons why I have rarely been seduced by faddy diets over the years – I love food too much. The very idea of beginning every meal with half a grapefruit or eating cabbage soup for days on end fills me with horror, but I have dabbled with others, most notably the Atkins diet, which focuses on a low-carb, high-fat and high-protein plan. This was prompted after watching a video Eamonn had taken of me while we were on holiday. When we got home, he connected the video recorder to the TV so we could look back on our first trip away with Jack, who was still a baby. There was the hotel. Oh, and our room. And look, there's the pool! I was watching it and then I thought, why is he filming that large woman dragging a sun lounger around the pool . . . and then the camera zoomed in, and I realised it was me. I was the large woman dragging the sun lounger.

OK, yes, I had just had a baby, although he was about five months old by this point, and yes, I was never going to be the person who would 'snap back' into her size 10 (make that size 12) jeans, but it was shocking to see. That wasn't how I looked in my head. I was caught off guard, oblivious to the camera, ungainly as I moved furniture around, and the truth was even more evident because I wasn't posing, holding my stomach in or covering up.

I couldn't believe Eamonn had filmed me looking so awful and that this was now captured for posterity, but he didn't see it that way. He didn't see *me* that way. He was filming because he thought it was funny how organised I was being with our loungers and the last thing he expected was for me to freak out about the way I looked.

It was a turning point, and I found the Atkins diet suited the way I ate because although I wasn't allowed bread and pasta (boo!), I could eat a lot of protein, like eggs and steak (yay!), which I loved. It worked and I lost a stone, feeling so much better in myself as well as being able to get back into my clothes. Over the years, if my jeans were feeling a little too snug or I was trying to be healthier, I stayed off the carbs for a while. It was the best way for me to shift a few pounds, but I never cared enough about being slim to diet for any length of time.

I am good at living life well and I find diets incredibly boring. Thanks to the menopause or age, or both, I now struggle with my weight. My old no-carbs trick doesn't work as well, and as tempting as those weight loss jabs are, I would prefer not to go down that road, although no judgement on those who have. One of the reasons I wouldn't is that I love cooking and eating and I don't want that to change. I even enjoy food shopping and prefer to walk around a supermarket than do an online order because I like to be inspired by the produce. I want to spend time with people who feel the same as me about a large glass of wine, a bowl of crisps or a wedge of cake.

I believe it's more important for me to tackle my shape and fitness and feel comfortable in my own skin than it is to obsess over my weight, and I try to stay away from the scales. That said, after a couple of sugar-free weeks where I exercised every day and was feeling good, I got on the scales. Oh, the agony. I had lost a pound. Just one single solitary bloody pound. Serves me right for stepping back on them when I know it's not about how much I weigh that matters. In fact, my Pilates instructor is threatening to take the scales off me because she says no good comes from getting on them.

For me, Pilates is the perfect exercise. I started doing it after Jack was born and I was on a mission to get back into shape. More importantly, I had a bad back, and after several trips to the chiropractor she said I was welcome to keep coming to her, but what I really needed to do was strengthen my core. She asked me if I had ever tried Pilates and suggested I go on to the Pilates Association website to find a registered instructor in my area. I looked it up and found two men and one woman, Siobhan, so I thought I would try her first. She sounded really nice on the phone and said she could come and teach me at home. When she asked for my address and we realised she lived one road away from me, it felt like it was meant to be.

I liked Siobhan straight away. She was fun, had great energy and was an amazing advert for the Pilates she taught. She could put her leg over her head. I mean, who wouldn't be impressed by that?! More to the point, she was hugely encouraging, and after a series of regular sessions of Classic Mat Pilates, I felt much fitter and my back was stronger.

Then life got in the way, and I let Pilates slide. It was harder to see Siobhan and by then she had opened a studio, so she was also incredibly busy, but we kept in touch. Recently, knowing I needed to do more than cut out pasta, I thought about taking up Pilates again. I don't like running, I rarely swim, yoga is a bit too slow for me and I am absolutely not a gym bunny, so this felt like the answer, and I messaged Siobhan. She invited me to the studio to try out Reformer Pilates, which is done on a machine with pulleys and springs, increasing resistance and making the exercises more effective. I was immediately hooked. Haha, little pun for you there!

I went to the studio regularly and occasionally Siobhan would come to me for a mat session. It was during one of these that I remembered I had a home Pilates machine tucked away in the garage. I know this is something you are unlikely to forget, but I'd bought it about five years previously and a lot had happened since then, as you all now know. It was one of my QVC purchases, on special offer at the time, and a couple of the presenters there had bought one and highly recommended it. I remember thinking it would be a good way to get back into Pilates, so I ordered it, and when it arrived I was determined that it wouldn't end up in the garage gathering dust, but I didn't have a clue how to use it, so unfortunately that was exactly what happened.

Siobhan and I got it out and brought it into the house. Now there is no excuse not to do something because it's right here, winking at me. I am trying to exercise most days, even if it's just for fifteen minutes before work. Doing little and often is better than big workouts once a week. I don't have to do hours on end, getting hot and sweaty, which I hate.

Like many of us, I have an image of how I think I look, so it's a surprise when I catch sight of myself in the mirror and realise I am not a tall willowy blonde! Yet Pilates has really changed my mindset and my shape. It makes me think of my body as a tree trunk, a solid and strong core, and all the branches – my limbs – can move around with better mobility.

I am not doing it to lose weight, I have chosen it to boost my suppleness, flexibility and strength. It has made me more aware of posture, and I am hopefully future-proofing against achy knees, which I can feel as I walk up and down stairs. Those joints aren't getting any younger!

Plus, I love the challenge of it. Can my leg do this? It can't yet but one day it may be able to, and I can already see improvement. Not only do I love it, but every time I feel I am progressing there is always an extension to the exercise or another level to reach, so it keeps me pushing myself and I can feel the physical and emotional difference. I am nervous to say out loud that I have found My Thing in case it tempts fate, but (whispers it) I think I have found my thing!

Siobhan sent me a quote recently that really resonated. I am not sure where it comes from, but it says: 'Be the oldest person in the Pilates class, not the youngest person in the nursing home.' That to me sums up where I am with my body and how I treat it.

Even though I hate physical elements of the ageing process, I am not in denial, nor am I trying to fight against it. I care about how I look but, more than that, I care about how I feel in my body. What I want now, as I hit my middle sixties, is to be strong, healthy and able to celebrate all the good parts of me, making the best of what I have. That's my mission for the years ahead. I know how fortunate I am to be here, to be working, to be curious about the future, and that's what I am prioritising. That is what matters.

11

At My Time of Life

I am so grateful to the many women, high profile and not, who have raised issues and campaigned for recognition, support and change around perimenopause diagnosis, hormone replacement therapy (HRT), menopausal symptoms and other related areas. One of the big strides forward has been to challenge society's attitude to it all, by which I mean the medical profession, our government and men, but also us women too. We need to be more vocal about our experiences, have a better understanding of what we are dealing with and keep this high on the agenda for those coming after us.

There were two moments that led me to believe I had hit the menopause. The first was one Christmas, maybe eight or nine years ago, and my mum was staying. I felt incredibly hot and rushed out of the back door, flapping at my top and relieved to be out in the freezing air. As I was standing outside thinking this was a bit weird, I had a sudden flashback to my mum doing a similar thing in our old house in Cornwall. My sister and I were watching TV, and she flew into the room complaining of how hot it was, and yanked the sash window up to let in the cold night air. She had hold of the hem of her jumper and was wafting it in an attempt to cool down. Exactly what I was doing in my back garden. Did this mean what I thought it meant?

Mum never talked about the menopause to me, or 'the change' as some people would mouth in a quiet, secretive way as if it was catching, although I do remember her often remarking how she was 'thickening up' around her waist.

The second prod to get checked out was more dramatic. At home, Jack had his own teenage den where he had a TV, PlayStation and his drum kit – somewhere his mates could come over to hang out without having to make small talk with me in the kitchen. It gave him a little independence while he was still under our roof, which I would have been ecstatic about at his age. He was very lucky to have it.

I was redecorating to make the room more appropriate for a teen and we were having a new carpet fitted. The day before it was due to arrive, I asked Jack if he could help me pack up his stuff and clear the room ready for the fitters. It was Sunday and neither of us wanted to do this, but we had no choice, and I wanted to get on with it so we were organised. I was filling boxes and chattering away until I became aware that Jack had gone quiet. He had been sorting through a pile of football magazines and was distracted, his head stuck in one of them. Several times I tried to get him to focus on the job in hand, calm and cajoling at first, but it wasn't working and he was moving at snail's pace through a pile of books.

My frustration was growing. I began to get annoyed, which sounded a lot like, 'Jack! I can't do all of this on my own!' He apologised, moved a couple of things and then slowed down again. I kept thinking of how lucky he was to have such a lovely room and how ungrateful he was not to be helping and, from nowhere, the rage came. He was perched on the edge of the sofa, idly flicking through another magazine, and I saw red.

I went up to him and yelled in his face, something like, 'I do everything for you! All I am asking for is a little bit of help! You know what, Jack? You are a spoilt little shit! I don't care about your carpet. Sort the room out yourself or don't.' Then I ran out of the room, slamming the door so hard I'm surprised it didn't come off its hinges.

I ran upstairs, threw myself on my bed and burst into tears. What on earth had just happened there? I was not proud of my behaviour. I had lost my temper, sworn at him and stormed off in a state. How did we get here? I calmed myself down, splashed water on my face and thought, I need to go back and sort this mess out.

Jack was sitting in exactly the same place I had left him, albeit looking a little shell-shocked. I don't think he could quite believe what had just happened either. In the midst of my astonishment about my reaction, I knew not to give a full-on apology. Certain facts remained. He was being lazy. I had asked him several times for his help. It was his room. He was lucky to have a new carpet.

I did the worst thing you should probably do in that situation. I just walked back in as if nothing had happened and continued to clear up, asking in a completely normal voice if there were books he wanted to keep. He played along with it and neither of us said anything about the awful scene.

A few days later, I was recounting the tale to a male friend of mine, making him laugh a lot about it in the retelling, and we were agreeing that it had been a hormonal outburst – and then he became serious.

'Oh Ruth, I think you should tell Jack about the menopause, because I was really worried about my mum,' he said.

'Yeah right, like I'm going to sit a fourteen-year-old boy down and tell him about the "change".' I wasn't comfortable with the idea.

'You must!' he insisted. 'Because exactly the same thing happened to me with my mum when I was a teenager and I told my friends I thought she was going mad.' He recounted the story. He told me he wasn't expected to do much around the house but the one job his mum had given him was to take the bin bag out. One day his mum came home from work, all sweetness and light, asking if he had had a lovely day, possibly ruffling his hair. You get the picture. And then she spied the bin bag, which he had forgotten to take out.

'Ruth, it was like watching *The Exorcist*. I swear her head swivelled on her neck and she screamed at me to take the bag outside. One minute she was fine, the next she was raging.' He shook his head in bewilderment at the memory of it. 'Soon after that, she sat me down and told me about this thing called the menopause. I am glad she told me because her behaviour then made total sense to me.'

My friend had made an important point. It felt so familiar to me. The moment where everything is fine, then it suddenly isn't and the fury bubbles up. A couple of days later, Jack and I were in the car together, which is always a good place for serious chats so you can both stare straight ahead and don't have to look at each other. I was not going to apologise because my basis for anger was justified, but I did need to tackle the way I had exploded.

'So Jack, I wanted to talk to you about the other day when I got a bit cross,' I began.

'A bit?' he said. 'That's an understatement.'

'Yes, well, I'm not apologising for telling you off, because I asked for your help several times. I just want to explain why my response was so extreme. There is something called the menopause. I don't know if they've covered it in PSHE?' I looked across at him for confirmation.

'I don't know,' he shrugged.

I took a deep breath and told him what I thought it would be useful for him to know without going into gory detail, focusing on hormones and getting an anger that it's hard to control.

'So, I am explaining this to you. I'm not apologising for telling you off, but I am sorry that it was so dramatic. And the bit where I shouted in your face and called you a spoilt little shit? That was totally uncalled for. I am really sorry. As you know, I don't normally behave like that.' It felt good to face into it.

'That's OK,' he said, and neither of us spoke for a moment.

'Anyway,' I said, 'your carpet's nice, isn't it!'

It struck me as completely unfair that for those of us who have had children later in life, menopause arrives as we are dealing with teenagers and elderly parents. It's what they call the Sandwich Generation. We are working full time, running a household, navigating teen angst and looking after or out for our parents – and all the while, our minds are trying to catch us out with brain fog, tiredness and fury. Sometimes our bodies are overwhelmed by waves of heat that begin at our toes and travel up through our body to explode out of the top of our head. How are we supposed to take a reasoned, logical view of things while all of this is happening?! Particularly when our teens may be behaving like little brats.

Sometimes, it isn't the hormones that get us, it's the real-life stuff, and there is no excusing that away. You know, the part where you are angry and everyone around you talks condescendingly about it being your hormones and then you say, 'NO, I JUST WANT SOMEONE OTHER THAN ME TO EMPTY THE BLOODY DISHWASHER FOR ONCE.' I don't call that menopause, I call that being annoyed.

A friend's husband once asked her how long the menopause lasted. Her response? 'I'm not sure, but I guess it lasts about as long as grumpy old man syndrome.'

Anyway, after Carpetgate, I thought I needed to go and talk to a medical professional to find out what I was dealing with. Full disclosure: I was fortunate enough to go privately to a hormone specialist for a menopause consultation, which was incredibly helpful. I had a blood test to find out where I was on the sliding hormonal scale, and I explained how flat I was feeling. While I was relieved not to have the brain fog other women I knew were experiencing, I had lost my mojo and I seemed to be lethargic all the time. It was hard to describe. Sometimes I thought I would cry, and I didn't know why.

Other times, I overreacted and could be incensed at the slightest thing. Like a teenager.

My blood test results showed my testosterone was so low it was hardly registering, and I was given bioidentical hormones. Within a week I could feel the difference, and I still take them now. I don't want to stop unless somebody says I should. Why would I come off them if they make me feel good?

I know women who have surfed the menopausal wave on little more than St John's Wort, and if that works for them then that's great. Some women don't want HRT or are not allowed to take it. It's a very personal decision and each of us has a different combination of symptoms so there is no one answer. The point is to try to find what works best for you. Now, with hormone replacement, Pilates and a sensible eating plan, I feel like I might be coming out the other side.

12

Sister, Dear Sister

As I move into this new phase of my life, I'm doing so without a lot of people. Particularly my adored Julia. She still is my big sister, although I am now older than she was when she died. She will be forever sixty-two. Just because she isn't here, it doesn't make her disappear. I have a lifetime of memories of her, and I carry her in my head, as well as finding any excuse to talk about her as often as I can.

I find it hard to say Julia 'battled' or 'struggled with' depression for many years because I don't think any of us really knew how impossibly hard it was for her or how she truly felt. Unless you have experienced it or live with someone with severe depression, it is difficult to imagine what it's like. I have had days when I've felt low, sad or anxious, but I know at my worst it was still so very far from what my sister lived with every day. I have never felt so desperate that I wouldn't want to be here anymore and that I couldn't share the terror of those thoughts. It must be the loneliest, bleakest place to be.

When we were young and went away to boarding school together, Julia took the responsibility of keeping an eye on me very seriously, as she did everything. She was only ten, but she had her feisty seven-year-old sister to look out for while our parents were in another country. I never considered what this must have been like for her until I was an adult.

Julia would come to my common room and check on me. She did it with such concern and care, she never played the bossy big sister role. When she turned up and asked for me, one of the girls would come and find me and, to my friends, I would huff and roll my eyes at being interrupted, but I never let her see that. I knew she was doing it out of love and duty.

Years later, when we were reminiscing about boarding school days with our parents, Dad said had either of us been unhappy he would have taken us out immediately. I said I had loved my time there, but my sister's response was quite different.

'I didn't like it, Daddy, but when you asked me if I was happy or if I wanted to come home, I said I was fine when what I really wanted to say was no, I am not happy. I hate it. I wanted to beg you to come and get me, but I didn't.' I think when she was a child, Julia said what she thought Dad wanted to hear, and I think she was worried that if they took her out of the school I would have to come too and then she would ruin it for me. My sister did what she perceived to be the right thing. She was always a people-pleaser, but I think that was exactly the point where she took on what I called the Cloak of Responsibility. I believe she wore it for the rest of her life.

As we grew up, Julia was always the sensible one. She was the kindest and most gentle soul you could hope to meet, and I knew how lucky I was to have her as a big sister. My first proper inkling that she had down times was when I was living in

Plymouth and she had got married and moved to Sussex. We were catching up over the phone, and I asked her what she was doing at the weekend. She gave the biggest sigh and said they were going out to choose a new sofa. She said it as if it was a difficult chore, like clearing the drains or defrosting the freezer. She went into detail about how worried she was, having to decide on a shape and colour. She could have been telling me she was going to the dentist for root canal treatment. At the time, I was in my little house, sitting on my grandma's old sofa because I couldn't afford a new one, and I was amazed that Julia wasn't thrilled about the prospect of shopping for a new couch. I would be ecstatic. It gave me an uncomfortable insight into her state of mind.

Over the years, I realised how hard it could be for her to make decisions, even when we were out shopping together for something inconsequential. She might be looking for the simplest thing – a black polo-neck jumper, say – and she found it impossible to choose. I couldn't understand it. How hard could it be, because surely a black polo neck was just a black polo neck? There were also times of joy that she couldn't seem to access, and I would chivvy her along, bemused by her lacklustre response. We were very different people, but we were incredibly close. I can't pinpoint the moment I knew she had severe depression, it was more of a growing understanding.

Julia was seeing the GP and had been on medication, but I wasn't living near her, so all I knew was what she allowed me to know and what my gut instinct told me. I can only speak from my own viewpoint, not from that of her husband, daughter and friends. After a particularly tough period, she seemed to be doing better and was upbeat and present for several years, so what happened next was a complete shock to me. I received the worst phone call I have ever had. My darling sister had taken her own life.

The next couple of hours were a total blur. I must have been wailing because Jack, my then sweet-sixteen-year-old son, was suddenly there with his arms around me and was hugging tightly. Perhaps he took the phone out of my hand. I don't remember what happened, but I will never forget the feeling of devastation that overwhelmed me. I thought about Julia, her husband, her daughter, and then I thought, oh God, my poor mum. She still didn't know.

Eamonn was away in Belfast at the time. Jack called him and I could hear him telling his dad not to worry and that he was with me. Eamonn was trying to book the earliest return flight he could, but he knew he wouldn't be able to get back that night, so he called Rylan, a close friend of ours, and told him what had happened. Eamonn asked if Rylan could call me and keep me talking so that he could get in touch with my girlfriends and see if they could get over to me. I don't remember much of that conversation with Rylan, but I just knew he was there and I will be forever grateful for that phone call.

Suddenly, there were Lucy and Louise on the doorstep – they had raced over, even though it was late. Lucy told me much later that she had been out for the evening and had had a few drinks, so she had to ask her daughter to drive her over. Eamonn had also rung Sam; she had switched her phone off and gone to bed, but when she checked it early the next morning she immediately jumped in the car and drove up from Salisbury. My three amazing friends formed a protective, loving circle around me.

There was no way I could give Mum the news over the phone, but no sooner had Sam arrived the next morning than she offered to drive me down to Sussex. Jack wanted to come with me. It was the worst journey of my life. I felt sick and numb, staring out of the window without seeing anything. Mum was not expecting us, but I couldn't risk calling her beforehand because I was liable to break down the minute I heard her voice.

We pulled into her drive, and I saw her stand up to see who had arrived. She spotted me and waved, breaking into a big smile, and came to the door. 'What a lovely surprise,' she said, just before I had to break her heart. Oh Mum, I thought, how do I tell you? How do I ever speak this? 'Oh Mum,' I blurted out, 'I have some terrible news.'

I still look back at this now and wonder if I did it in the right way, but then how do you ever know what the right way is? I told Mum that Julia had died but I couldn't quite bring myself to say how, thinking that it was too much to take in in one go. I remember her legs buckling – I thought she was going to collapse or die in front of me from the shock – and Jack caught hold of her and helped her into the sitting room. I was an absolute mess, and I kept trying to pull myself together. Yes, this was my sister, but this was my mum's child. Her first baby.

Jack went and made tea and the two of us looked at each other, mirroring the shock and anguish. I didn't want it to be true. I didn't want to be sitting here talking to my mum about her worst nightmare. All I could think was that we were never going to see Julia again, never be able to call her or go out together. It was too big and devastating to contemplate.

I said to Mum, 'I am taking you home with me. Let's pack a bag.' It wasn't until we unpacked at my house that we realised we had a pyjama top without bottoms, one slipper and no toothbrush. It was clear that we were attempting a simple task while we were completely traumatised.

Back at home, Sam stayed, making cups of tea and preparing meals that she encouraged us to try to eat. Eamonn had managed to book on to a flight but wouldn't be back until the following day. I don't think I slept that night and early in the morning I saw the light was on in Mum's room, so I made us both a cup of tea and took them in. I lay down next to her and we stared at the ceiling. 'Why?' Mum whispered. 'Why didn't she talk to us?' 'I don't know, Mum,' I said. 'I don't know.'

The biggest unanswered questions that ricochet around my head – and will forever – are: Why did she take her own life? Why didn't she talk to me about how she was feeling? Why did I not know she felt like that? Why? Why? Why? I could carry the guilt forever, if I could just have an idea of why she did it. And then from confusion came the anger. How could she? How could she do this to the people she loved most in the world? And then I fell into the deepest well of sadness.

When Eamonn came home, he immediately swept me up and took me into another room before seeing everyone else and I sobbed in his arms. Weirdly, I remember worrying that I was getting mascara on his shirt. While this was awful for us, what about Julia's husband and daughter? I couldn't contemplate their pain.

At Julia's funeral, which was full to the rafters with her friends as well as us family, I was determined to do a reading for her as she had done for our dad. It was incredibly hard, but the memory of her strength got me through it. My voice broke at the end, and I looked up to see my three friends willing me on. Sitting in the pew, my shoulders heaving with silent sobs, Jack put his arm around me and I thought how hard it must be for him to see me like this. We held the wake at the same lovely hotel we had been at for Dad's, and the family and I put together a big photo collage of Julia as she had done for our dad. I still have the picture boards in my office, but I can't bring myself to look at them yet.

In the immediate aftermath of Julia's death, I would wake up each morning and for a few seconds, all was right with the world – and then reality hit me square in the jaw. Oh God, my sister has killed herself. Oh my God, my poor mum is next door. I took time off work but eventually I knew that I needed some structure back and a reason to get out of bed and wash my hair in the morning. I was ready to get out of the house.

When I went back to *Loose Women*, they couldn't have been more supportive. On air, they were ready to step in if I needed a break or felt I couldn't continue. The same at *This Morning*. I had just returned, and we were hosting a phone-in when a caller talked about depression. I could feel the tears coming and the director asked if I was OK. I shook my head, and he told the camera to stay on Eamonn while I slipped off and he told the viewers, who knew about Julia, that I just needed a moment.

Incredible support all round and without it I would have broken into a million tiny little pieces.

Some find other people's grief hard to deal with, particularly those who have never experienced it. They don't know how to react or what to say and it is easier for them to cross the road or avoid you when they see you coming. It's brutal, but it makes the people who face into it with you all the more special.

Had Julia told me what she was planning to do, I would have been so shocked, but I believed I could have stopped her. I believed that for quite some time, but I know this is unlikely to be the case, because if she had wanted saving, I think she would have shared more. In listening to other people's stories over the years, I know that when someone has made the decision that they don't want to be here anymore, unless they choose to tell someone, then they often find a way to leave.

Whenever I hear about somebody who has taken their own life, I immediately think of their poor family and what it will do to the loved ones they leave behind because I know what they are going through. Like a grenade thrown into the middle of my family, the shock waves spread to my lovely Uncle Arthur and Auntie Rosa. Seeing them at Julia's funeral, smartly dressed and absolutely broken, was enough to make me sob. The waves of grief that follow loss can threaten to drown us all at points. I am here to tell you they won't, but it doesn't feel like that at the time.

I knew Julia had bouts of depression over the years, and she had a particularly awful episode a few years before she died, but we had talked a lot, and I thought I could help her fix it. Me, the problem-solver, who as soon as someone presented me with an issue was then driven to find an answer. I was sure I could do the same for my sister. How wrong I was.

It reminded me of a story Mum used to tell, about the time we lived in Oxford, and she heard a commotion outside. She looked out of the window and there I was, at around five years old, with Julia, who was about seven, and her friend. They were both standing behind me and I was squaring up to the local bully. I had my fists up in fight position and I was shouting, 'Come on then!' and 'Leave my sister alone!' Mum had to come out and break it up. I would get into scrapes to protect Julia and now I felt that for all the little battles we had won together, we had lost the war.

A while ago, too late to be of any use to Julia, I heard an interview with Stephen Fry, talking about depression. He said that, sometimes, when someone talks to you about how low they are feeling, they aren't looking for a solution, they just want you to listen. That was incredibly powerful to hear, a sucker punch to my gut, because I realised I was always offering Julia solutions, bouncing around with my latest suggestion for how she could be happier. What if she had felt under pressure from me? Did I add to her anxiety by telling her I had read something about yoga being good for depression? Or I had found a retreat, and I was going to send her a pamphlet or a link? And did I compound it, the next time I spoke to her, by asking if she had followed up on the thing I had mentioned? Listening to Stephen talking was like somebody had switched on a light and suddenly my relationship with Julia was illuminated. While I desperately wanted her to be happy, I think I was also scared she would leave us all and if I could try to fix her, that meant we could keep her here for longer.

How tedious it must have been for her to hear me banging on about the latest thing to ease the blues or frighten away the Black Dog. Julia, do this and you will be cured! OK, in fairness to myself, I wasn't that insensitive, and I was doing it from a place of unconditional and bottomless love, but I realise now that in trying to help I was just putting pressure on her. And every time she didn't do what I had suggested, did she feel like she had let me down? Did she think we were all fed up with her? Awful, awful, awful, and no answers, really, other than the glimmers I glean from listening to other people's experiences. Finding those who understood and empathised with what I was going through really helped me when it was impossible to make sense of it all. I am not sure I will ever be able to make sense of it, but I am learning to live alongside it.

Julia had a lovely husband, a beloved daughter and good friends, and she seemed happy in her career as a gardener. It was hard to see from the outside what had gone so wrong, but I know that's not how depression works. Sometimes she would spiral and I couldn't work out what the trigger was, then other times, when cataclysmic things happened like our dad dying, she had the strength to cope with it, much more than I did. I would worry about what it was that would affect her without ever being able to work it out. Maybe she didn't know herself. Maybe it had nothing to do with me. Maybe that's a couple of answers right there.

I always wear the bracelet I gave Julia when she was my bridesmaid. It's something of hers that connects us. Now it is just me and Mum from our original family unit of four. Sibling relationships are supposed to be the longest ones we have, and I never contemplated a future without her – and my mum never thought she would outlive her child.

Here is what I want you to know and remember about my sister, Julia: not about how she died, but how she lived. She was smart, creative and amazing. She couldn't see it and was uncomfortable with compliments, but I told her all the time how great she was. She was the most fantastic cook and baked the best cakes. Whenever I smell Clinique Aromatics now, it reminds me of her because it was her favourite perfume. She was an intuitive gardener. She was curious, clever, funny and self-deprecating, often to her detriment. She was part of a women's swimming club and the sailing club and made great friends at both. She was a loving daughter, sister, wife and a devoted mother.

I think of her all the time and I wish, wish, wish she was here, but I now understand that she didn't want to be and I respect that. It's taken me a long time to feel like that. I miss her and the sisterly relationship we had, but now the memories make me smile more than they bring tears. I hope she is happy, wherever she is. I like to imagine she is with our dad, sailing somewhere sunny and warm.

Talking about her really helps and my counsellor friend Jill told me to make sure I didn't lock Julia in a box. Mum and I shared memories and looked at photos before her dementia made that too difficult. The world was a much better place with my sister in it and I could cry about her loss every day, but I know she wouldn't want that for me. I made a silent promise to us both that I would try to live the best and happiest life I can in her memory.

13

Loose Women, Lovely Friends

Never underestimate the power of friendship, particularly the female kind. I doubt I need to tell you this, but I want to acknowledge here what a steadying presence it has been throughout my life. I can't imagine how I would have navigated the difficult times without my friends – and luckily, I don't have to think about it, because they are always there for me, as I hope I am for them.

I don't have a big circle of friends. I have those that I have been close to since childhood, work colleagues who have become great mates, and lovely acquaintances picked up over the years, male and female. My friends have been there for me in my darkest times, particularly in the last ten years or so when I lost my dad, followed by my sister, and then my marriage broke up. That was when I needed the sisterhood more than ever.

I talked to women who had been through the same and they shared their distress, how they dealt with it and the belief that if they were OK, I would be too. When people share their painful experiences with such vulnerability, it is generous of them and invaluable to you. I was so grateful and relieved to see how they were thriving in their new lives. They hadn't broken.

My friends called me early in the morning, late at night, they let me talk, they came round, they brought me food, and they kept me going. They encouraged me to go out, they fed me shepherd's pie, they sat on the sofa watching telly with me, they handed me tissues and hugged me tight when I had a good cry.

Not only do I have a wonderful group of friends, I am also one of the anchor presenters in the well-known band of merry women on ITV's *Loose Women*, a brilliant community I have been part of for over twenty-six years. Can you believe that? I can't. Where does the time go?! The programme is older than my son and there are not many TV shows that run for that long. It has gone by in a heartbeat, and I have loved every second of it. I am one of its biggest fans and most vocal cheerleaders – I guess I would say that, yet whether I was part of it or not, I would watch because there is something incredibly powerful in seeing a group of women on screen.

I was fascinated by the idea of the programme when I was asked to do the pilot. It was a genius concept. There had never been any kind of all-female chat show or panel discussion and I was so proud to be a small part of it. The title didn't convince me at first because I immediately thought of 'loose' in terms of morals, which felt a bit regressive, but when put into the context of plain speaking and opinions – loose-lipped, if you will – it made sense. I think it still suits the show really well.

I love the line-up of women – an often-changing cast of familiar characters – and how no two days are ever the same, even though the format remains set. It's a dynamic show that continues to evolve and move with the times. I always say that if you gave four panellists a topic to discuss on Monday and the following day gave the same subject to four other panellists, the views could be completely different, which is the essence of the show.

The programme doesn't belong to one group of women, it's a chorus of us who dip in and out depending on professional commitments and domestic situations, with some taking time away to go off and do something else, like act in a play or have a baby. It reflects life. There are several generations brought together, listening to each other, sharing our opinions and learning. If someone is more informed than me or has a strong view about something, I come to the conversation with an open mind. There may be an angle I haven't thought about or something I may not agree with, but they can change my perception. I have learned so much from the women I've worked with.

Can I dispel the myth, once and for all, that the presenters on *Loose Women* hate each other and the rumour that while it may be smiles and hugs in front of the camera, it's handbags at dawn behind the scenes? It's absolutely not true! There is a running commentary in the press about the various fall-outs and feuds, which, to my knowledge, have never happened. Maybe there is an assumption that because we are an all-female line-up, once the cameras are off it's a bitchy gossip fest of women fighting each other. This is a familiar but derogatory and offensive attitude.

We have built many friendships among the group. Of course, there are always people you get on better with than others, but there isn't a single woman I wouldn't want to be on the panel with. Hand on heart. In all the years I have been working on the show, I have never said to the production team that there is someone I want to avoid. It's a bit like going out for dinner with a group of friends and knowing that it doesn't matter who you sit next to at the table because you will always have a good time.

There are a few women who have become closer friends, like Coleen Nolan. Coleen and I are very different people, and we didn't know each other before we worked together on the show. We clicked instantly, although we weren't immediate best mates, and the relationship developed from there. I love sitting on the panel with her and hearing her take on things. She is one of the funniest people I know, and we have excellent banter, sometimes ending up in the press with one of our witty retorts rebranded as 'rude' or a jokey moment of pretending to leave the studio termed 'storming off'. We just laugh about it.

Coleen is incredibly intuitive and always knows if there is something wrong with me. She can also defuse a difficult topic with the nimbleness of a bomb disposal expert. If we are in the heat of the discussion and need to move on, Coleen often has an appropriate quip or a good one-liner to sign off on. That's not to say that she is the only loose woman for me! I could list so many of them, including Janet Street-Porter, who is so utterly and brilliantly herself, and Jane Moore, who is whip-smart and a woman's woman through and through. Whether I have worked with someone for ten years or ten minutes, if they have joined the *Loose Women* gang then I just know I will like them.

As one of the anchors, sitting at the end of the panel, I don't see my role as more important than anyone else's. The only difference is that I am aware of timings and going into a break, plus I do the links, which I really enjoy. There is complete equality among us. We are a genuine, supportive bunch who have been there for each other through very difficult periods including divorce and death, as well as the joyous times of babies, marriage and exciting work opportunities.

The mix of generations works brilliantly because I feel that we learn from each other. I think it helps our younger colleagues too, even when we talk about stuff like the menopause or ageing parents, because it gives them an understanding of what is to come. In return, they share what it's like to be dating or starting a family in these times of social media and cancel culture, something the elders of the team have less experience with.

In the morning, when we arrive for the show, there will be a meeting with that day's panellists and the production team. We drink our tea or coffee and spend the first ten minutes catching up on how everyone is, what we may have watched on telly and any big life updates. Sometimes there will be women who I haven't worked with for a while and it's always a treat to be together and give each other the lowdown on life.

The producer calls order and outlines the potential topics we could cover that day. We look at the top news stories, trending subjects and anything we may personally feel strongly about. We all have a say in what is included. It can create a discussion and if two women disagree this is likely to make it to the screen because who wants to watch us all agreeing with each other? We aren't an echo chamber. We love a fierce debate, but we respect opposing views and we don't fall out about it. There is always a fun element to give light to the shade.

It would be fascinating to go back to some of our early shows and see what we were talking about then. What were we focused on at the turn of the century and the start of a new millennium? The misconception among those who have not watched the show at some point in the last twenty-six years is that we talk about make-up, hairstyles and shoes. There can be this assumption that a group of women will automatically do this and yes, there are those conversations, but they are rare as the main thrust of each day focuses on more serious issues like world news, current affairs and things we feel passionate about.

We have an idea of what we are covering before we go on air and we have plotted out the time to fit with the commercial breaks and the guest joining us later in the programme, but I love those times when our discussion takes a different turn from the one we had in the meeting. That's what makes the live show so special and fresh, because it's honest conversation. It's not scripted, and it gives us each the opportunity to speak while making us all great listeners. Our reactions are genuine and unstaged. It's one of the reasons why I think the team are so good at what they do and why the show is still going after all this time.

We are in a circle of trust that begins outside the studio and continues live on air. Sometimes we talk to each other about personal stuff that we are not going to be public about so we are careful around that topic on the show. Everyone knows if one of us is going through something that we are not prepared to talk about yet, it remains sacrosanct, and we have each other's backs. I can't tell you what a wonderful feeling that is because we are not just work colleagues, we are friends. That includes the excellent mixed-gender production team too. They are part of the hallowed private space, and we all hear stuff that doesn't leave the room. A lot of our conversations don't get on air. We protect each other, not just the women, but the men too.

I was boosted by their support when I went back to work after my sister died. I had taken some time out and when I returned, I knew I was safe there and that I wouldn't be expected to talk about anything triggering. Then, when I was going through my marriage separation, I took some time out before the news was made public.

Going back to *Loose Women* after that felt like walking into safe, open arms. Nobody made a big deal of me being there because they knew I was trying to hold it together; they just welcomed me like I had come home after a trip away. Live on air, back on the panel in my happy place, I did my usual opening and then Coleen interrupted, 'Can I just say, before we go on, it's so good to have you back.' There was huge spontaneous applause from the audience, and I wanted to cry, but I managed not to, and we moved on to the topics of the day.

All of us have shit happening. You, me, everybody. Being someone off the telly doesn't protect me from any of it. When I am on *Loose Women* my hair and make-up may be done and I've got nice clothes on, which is a treat, but I am still me, dealing with life. The great thing about being there is that I am surrounded by a community of friends, and I do not feel alone for a moment. Whatever each of us may be going through, it's likely it has already been experienced by another one of the group and production team.

Loose Women directly reflects the relationship I have with my own friends. In my personal life I love the Friday night catch-ups with girlfriends, opening a couple of bottles of wine, getting snacks out and no conversation is off limits unless someone gives us the nod to avoid an issue. As everyone arrives, we say how lovely the other one looks, followed by all of us saying our clothes are too tight, or we didn't do much exercise that week or we look really tired. It's amazing how easily we can criticise ourselves. Self-deprecation can easily switch from being jokey to something more serious, digging away at our confidence. We can be our own worst enemy, so this is where friends step in to lift our heads from our navels and demand we stop beating ourselves up.

I've already said that I need to make a conscious effort to say yes to nice things because I can easily talk myself out of leaving the house. That's not to say I am not social, because I see my friends a lot – it's just that we sit in each other's kitchens instead of wine bars. One of us may say, 'Sorry, I'm not changing later, I'll just be in my slobs', meaning comfortable, relaxed clothing, and someone else will reply, 'Oh God, me too' and another might add, 'And I haven't washed my hair for several days' and we all say, 'Don't worry, it's just us.' None of us cares. The downside of this is that we have very few photos of each other that could be considered Instagram worthy because we are always in our slobs.

We order a curry so nobody has to cook and then we get down to it, talking about work, kids and family. How's your dad doing? Did your daughter get that job? How are the hot flushes? Did you see that documentary everyone is talking about? We laugh a lot and at least one person cries before the end of the evening, which often sets the rest of us off.

We do talk about relationships, particularly if someone is going through a break-up or has met a new squeeze, but we don't spend nearly as much time talking about men as they think we do! Neither are we men-haters! We can sometimes be accused of this on *Loose Women*, which is frustrating because it's not the case. Why can't women hang out together without the assumption that it is because we want to moan about men?! Also, we know our male viewers benefit from our discussions and gain insight into our world because they have told us, particularly when we talk about periods, childbirth and the menopause. We know they take notice, because this is happening to their wife, sister or female friends.

As on *Loose Women*, in the comfort of our homes, among our friends, a topic may come up that a couple of us feel very strongly about and we share opinions, sometimes changing someone's mind or giving them pause for thought. Then there are those times when a subject hits home for some and not others. I don't need to have a view on everything, and I enjoy sitting back and listening to others who know more than me, whether it's at the end of the *Loose Women* desk or at my dining table. It's so stimulating, even if I am an observer.

Now, I couldn't write this chapter on friendship without shoehorning in a mention of my adored Maggie, because a dog is a girl's best friend. She is rather old, a bit deaf and doddery, but she is still my dearest companion. I can tell her anything. If I feel overwhelmed or stressed, I take her out for a walk and watch her snuffling around in the grass and enjoying the attention of passers-by. I try not to go on my phone as we wander so I can be completely in the moment, as she always is.

I love seeing Maggie with my mum, too, and often take her to visit. I think dogs are really intuitive. When Mum broke her hip the first time, she was still living in her bungalow, so she came to stay with me to recuperate. Every night I asked Mum if she was ready to go up to bed and we would go upstairs to find Maggie was ahead of us and waiting outside Mum's bedroom door. I always helped Mum into bed and then lifted Maggie up, and she snuggled down next to her. She usually sleeps with me, but it was like she knew Mum needed company. Mum's need was greater than mine and I like to think Maggie was watching over her.

I could not have got through many things in my life without my friends (and Maggie!). They have been the wind beneath my wings, my sisterhood and my scaffolding. I sincerely hope I continue to be the same for them. The fact is that we don't need loads of friends, we just need those few who really get us, who turn up at the worst times and show their love quietly and unconditionally. The friends who we most want to crash on the sofa with in front of the telly and watch *Strictly Come Dancing* together. The friends who we love and are proud of, who we would drop anything for and who do the same for us. The friends we most want to celebrate and celebrate with.

Priceless, precious and always there with a pep talk, these friendships remain with you throughout your life and no matter what happens in work, family and health, they are unfailing. Let's raise a large gin and tonic to our mates. Here's to women supporting women, to female and male friendship and to laughing until tea comes out of our nostrils. Even in my darkest times, my friends are the people who remind me who I am, that I can survive anything – and they make me feel fabulous.

14

Fashionista

At *Loose Women* we have several amazing stylists who organise our on-screen wardrobes. They know exactly what I am most comfortable wearing, like a suit, and what my pet hates are, including above-the-knee skirts. I don't go for flim-flam floaty blouses, as I call them, because they are hard to attach a microphone to, unlike a blazer, which is one of my favourite things to wear, particularly as it covers my middle.

When I think back to my teenage years, I thank goodness that camera phones weren't yet invented because all the fashion faux pas I made back then are lost in the mists of time. We didn't take many photos as it was expensive to get them developed and I certainly wouldn't have thought of taking them of myself. I had an eye on fashion, like every teenager, and dressed in 'Oxford bags' trousers and shoes with thick crepe soles – a popular choice at the time. I always had a pretty good awareness of what suited me, and I wasn't seduced by the latest look if it didn't work for me.

One of the trends I did buy into was the grandad shirt and I made my own by cutting the collars off my dad's old shirts. This, cinched in with a belt and worn with Levi jeans tucked into a pair of cowboy boots, and I was good to go. I would customise clothes too, adding strips of patterned fabric to the inside of a jacket cuff so when I rolled it back there was a flash of colour. I always loved sewing and knew how to choose the right material, cut out patterns and create a skirt or top.

Making my own clothes and adapting things put me in tune with my body shape and gave me an early understanding of cut and style. I wasn't really swayed by magazines, famous people or my contemporaries. Nor did I go rogue in the manner of a fashion student and plunder the local charity shops, although I loved a jumble sale and would often find something there that I could unpick and transform, usually attracted first by the fabric.

Over the years, I have had to pay attention to my wardrobe because I am on the telly. It's an enjoyable part of the job, but not something I've given much time or thought to because I am lucky enough to work with stylists who do it for me. I turn up for TV shows, magazine shoots or before an event and there is a team of hair, make-up and wardrobe experts ready to swoop, like a squad of fairy godmothers, buffing me into something half decent and always with great conversation. If you see me looking good, then that's usually with the help of them. They say it takes a village!

Funny, then, that I find myself with a foot in the fashion industry in what may seem like a left-field move and yet, when I look back to my youth and my needlework O level, it makes me smile.

About five years ago, out of the blue, the legendary shopping channel QVC got in touch. I was in the ITV canteen with my agent, catching up on work stuff, and she said QVC were keen to meet me for a chat. She wasn't sure what they wanted but they'd asked if I would meet them for a coffee. I already liked QVC and had bought things from them, so I knew what they did and felt honoured that they were interested in me.

'That's amazing!' I was astounded.

'I am so glad you said that,' said my agent, 'because some people can be a bit funny about shopping channels.'

'Not me,' I said cheerily.

Cut to a meeting at QVC with the heads of various departments, including fashion and homeware. There was a bit of general chit-chat, they showed me around the studios and told me more about the channel, but nothing specific was mentioned. Afterwards, I didn't hear from them so I put it to the back of my mind until my agent called and said QVC had been back in touch and would I be interested in working with them to create my own fashion range?

I had never thought about designing clothes, but as soon as it was mentioned, although it took me by surprise, I was absolutely thrilled with the idea. Over the years I have learned to trust my gut reaction and my dad's words are often in my head, reminding me: 'What is the worst that can happen, Ruthiee?' Well, not much in this instance, Dad.

I gave a resounding yes to what has turned out to be a long, fruitful, busy and wonderful relationship with the channel. I'm a very hard worker, but I have to love something and be sure about it to give it my all. Had someone asked if I would like to learn to play golf, I would have said nah, you're all right thanks, but it was impossible to say no to this opportunity to have my own label with all the expertise and support that comes from QVC. Sometimes, things come into your life that you don't expect or don't always immediately recognise as right for you, but taking a leap of faith and being rewarded for that is such an amazing feeling.

I knew I had a lot to learn, and I am still learning all these years later, but I didn't doubt my decision then and I still don't, which must mean I made the right one. I already knew of my co-host, Jackie Kabler, because I remembered her from her reporter days on GMTV, where she was great and always looked incredibly stylish. Jackie was very kind to me when I started at QVC, showing me the ropes, but she couldn't believe how nervous I was on our first show, considering the hours and hours of live telly I had already clocked up. Yet this was a different genre, and QVC was new to me. It was important that it went well, not just for my own sense of pride but for the channel that had put its faith in me.

On that first show, I was more nervous than I had been in a long time. I always have a little buzz of adrenaline before any live telly, and I think this is good because it keeps me on my toes. It reminds me to pay attention, listen, learn, be ready to pivot if something changes, and it stops me getting complacent. I never think, I've got this or can switch on autopilot, because if you relax then that is likely to be the exact point where something will go wrong. The QVC presenters are fantastic and brilliant at what they do. I would challenge even the best TV presenters to come and do a stint on the channel because it really is a baptism of fire, with no script or autocue for two-hour live shows. It sharpens your senses, tests your reflexes and checks your stamina.

As well as putting myself out there on screen, I had the more significant pressure that I was introducing my own label. I am a TV presenter, that's my day job, and then here I was masquerading as a fashion designer. How would that go down? Imposter syndrome got me again!

I was about to reveal my range of clothes I had worked hard on for months, along with an expert team, and I had made decisions about styles, colours, cut, material and look.

There was a lot riding on this. QVC had manufactured a new line, and my name and reputation were pegged to it. What if women like me didn't like what I had done? What if nobody bought anything? It was like showing someone my baby for the first time and them wrinkling their nose in distaste, thinking it was ugly. I needn't have worried.

The beauty of working with QVC was that they positively encouraged the collaboration from every aspect. Yes, my name would help sell the clothes to women in my age group, but they also wanted my creative input, which I thank them for. When I first joined them, I decided to start as I meant to go on and was clear about what I loved to wear and, more importantly, what I hated. I knew I couldn't sell something if I wouldn't wear it myself and I had strong opinions about what I thought worked. QVC encouraged me to be open and confident with my feedback, but I also understood how little I knew about the business of fashion, including pattern cutting, production, marketing and sales. It has been a fascinating learning process with a great team of professionals and we respect each other's input and expertise. I adore every element of it.

To begin with, I was set on a neutral palette, a place I was always happiest with navy, black and camel, and I shied away from bright colours. In my day-to-day life, I stuck to a simple look with the odd bold scarf or bag chucked in for good measure. The team explained that the QVC woman loves colour and while we could make a line of T-shirts in classic tones, we also needed to add pink, lemon, apple green and maybe a lilac or purple. Apparently, pink was a best-selling colour, but I was hesitant because it was so opposite to what I wore. I trusted that QVC knew their stuff and sure enough, in my debut range the pink top sold out first.

Over the years, working with colour has encouraged me to embrace it myself. It doesn't mean I have to wear pink, but I am much more adventurous. I still wear a lot of camel and navy, but now I throw in pistachio green, chocolate brown and I am a big fan of orange. I bought myself the industry Pantone colour book (which was a bit of an investment, but worth it) and I refer to it regularly when I am designing. Every year the Pantone colour of the season is selected so we may incorporate it somewhere. We don't slavishly follow trends, but we are aware of them and include them if we like them.

If we have a discussion about a colour, design or style and I still absolutely hate it and would never wear it in a million years, then QVC respect that and don't push me to include it. I don't want anything out there with my name on it that I am not passionate about or can't see the point of.

Two years ago, QVC suggested I do a holiday range, and I jumped at the chance because I never felt I had nailed my holiday wardrobe, swimwear particularly. It reminded me of being away in Portugal one year. I was wearing a random bikini with a sarong that didn't match and a bag that didn't go with anything. I looked up to see a very elegant woman gliding to a sun lounger, head to toe in matching bikini and sarong with a bag in an accent colour. She looked amazing. I remember hating her in that moment, but not personally, I was just jealous. I wanted to be her.

A lot of ideas for my range come from these sorts of moments. My understanding of fashion has grown with QVC, and I know so much more about what my customer wants. The thing I am still getting my head around is working a year in advance. I am fascinated by how the team forecast trends: going to the shows, industry events, trade shows, interiors and even looking at the big movies coming up that will influence the catwalk. Then they take that knowledge and see it through the eyes of the QVC woman, understanding which elements of it will appeal to her while considering budget and practicalities.

We know what our ladies like because we ask for their feedback and they tell us, so if a colour or style proves unpopular, we ditch it. Often, this response comes in real time. When they message us, this sort of dynamic interaction is thrilling, particularly in the middle of a live show, and I make a note of what we discover as well as reading the reviews and responding. We see them all, good or bad, although luckily we don't have very much of the latter.

I very rarely have to shop for clothes anymore because I genuinely wear my own collection, it's not a PR stunt. The first time I realised I was head to toe in *Ruth Langsford* was one morning, as I was rushing out. I did a last check in the mirror and thought oh look, the scarf from my collection. Oh, and the jacket too. Plus, the jumper, jeans, boots and even the handbag. I promise I had not meant to do that. I dressed in what I loved, and it just happened to be all my own work!

When I am out and about and someone says to me, oh I love your top, I can say, thanks, it's one from my range. And so are the trainers, joggers and denim jacket that I'm wearing. Sometimes they're surprised that I'm wearing the clothes I design, like they expect me to be very distant from QVC and swanning around in expensive designer gear. I wear more items from my latest season, so it is in stock if someone loves it and wants to buy it, but I also wear a lot from previous years. My old faithfuls, which have lasted so well. We don't do throwaway fashion, it's about durability, does it wash well, will the colours hold?

This may sound a little big-headed, but when people ask me what's the inspiration behind my range, I say it is based on what I want to wear. It's as simple as that. If I like it, there may be other women who will like it too.

I don't think my look has changed significantly over the years. As I've said, I have never been a strict follower of trends and hated the pressure to look 'fashionable'. When I lived in the

West Country for many years, I would get nervous coming up to London because I wasn't sure what everyone was 'wearing in the city', which is a bit ridiculous now I come to write it down. I didn't need to be told what to wear, I knew what suited me and what made me feel good. Once I began to feel like this then all the pressure to be and look a certain way just disappeared and a sort of uniform emerged for me. I love blazers, longish jackets, well-cut jeans, boots with a heel and a nice top. How lucky am I to now be designing my own!

I've always said that I'm a team player, not a leader, but there have been moments at QVC where I have needed to step up and say what I think. I take advice but I also want to bring everyone on board with me and I know I need to use my voice and give my opinion. I am not shouty or bossy, but with age comes the absolute understanding of what I want. I am not saying I know everything, I am just saying I know what I like.

Considering I've stepped into an industry I have no previous experience in, I haven't once felt the old ghost of imposter syndrome hovering around since that first broadcast. I am very honest about how much I want to learn so there is no pretence about my ability, nor do I feel I have anything to prove, beyond being professional and doing a good job.

In one of the early design meetings, I said I wanted to make a good pair of jeans and there was a tumbleweed moment among the team because jeans are really difficult to get right. I knew that – I had often been reduced to tears trying to find a pair that fitted, were comfortable and that I liked. I was very specific about what I wanted. They needed to have stretch, be high-waisted so no muffin top, and I didn't want any gaping at the back. Is it possible, I asked the team. OK, let's try, was the response. We did and I now have the jeans of my dreams.

I hope this doesn't sound trite, but the label and the show have created a community of amazing women who watch us every week and update us on their life events. They aren't always there on the sofa ready to shop, and some even text in saying, 'I'm not shopping tonight, Ruth, because I can't afford it, but I am here to enjoy the show!' One woman messaged to say she was 'sitting on her hands' to stop herself using her credit card, which made us all laugh, and this phrase has now stuck. Everyone is welcome to watch, whether they are buying or sitting on their hands.

A big thrill for me is when women send in a photo of themselves wearing a piece from my collection and they have chosen it for a special occasion so I can see the confidence it has given them. On the live shows I am very honest, I talk about my flabby bits, how I hate my knees and I don't like the tops of my arms anymore, and I hope sharing this kind of vulnerability shows other women that none of us is perfect. Jackie and I always joke around about our body hang-ups, which is very reflective of female friendship where we banter but also bolster each other.

You can't please all of the people all of the time and I know some will look at my clothing range and say, 'Not for me, thank you.' That's totally fine and underlines the point I want to make about how we choose to look as we age. We need to find our own style and not be swayed by fashion, influenced by celebrity or think we are too old to wear something. Too old?! We can wear what the hell we want.

What is fashion, after all? It's just clothes. But they are a way for us to make ourselves feel happier, more confident and visible in middle age. I care less about what people think of me now than I ever have and this is the most empowering place to be, so what I wear is part of that. You put something on, and you want to feel great, look great and be comfortable, which is exactly my ethos. I don't want to grit my teeth and spend the day or evening in something tight or scratchy or faff around with fiddly buttons. Nor do I want to chase the latest trend that doesn't suit me or compare myself to other women and wish I looked like them. I am me. I know what I like.

Of course I want to look stylish with a nod to fashion, and I am not giving up on myself now I am in my mid-sixties, but I don't want to be awkward in an outfit. I want good-quality classics, not throwaway fashion. We often see ourselves differently from the way the world sees us, and we can be our own harshest critics, particularly when it comes to how we look. Ultimately, what we wear doesn't matter, it is how we feel in the clothes that counts, and we need to find that place of joy and try to have more fun with our wardrobe.

15

When Your Confidence Goes AWOL

I realise, as I have been writing this book, just how often a lack of confidence has slowed me down in the past or tried to stop me from being who I wanted to be. I wouldn't have said I struggled with being self-assured, and I doubt it's evident in public, but it has been a stumbling block at times, as it can be for so many of us. The liberating thing about where I am now in my life means I am grabbing confidence with both hands and not letting go – because if not now, then when? It has to be now!

My confidence has definitely grown with age. Like building a house, brick by brick, our experiences add to our ability, understanding and self-reliance. Yes, there are knockbacks, but I like to think that it doesn't take me long to return to myself now. It reminds me of one of those toys from my childhood that you knock over, they wobble but they get back up.

There are times when we lose our sense of self, maybe for moments or even for years. Our confidence dips or disappears. It feels easier, safer in fact, to stay at home. As a homebird, I know I could settle into that way of life and it is dangerous. We still need to step out of our comfort zone, not necessarily too far, but in a meaningful way, because this is the place we grow from.

When I suggest we can sometimes take a risk, I say this speaking as the most risk-averse person you are likely to meet.

While I am up for taking the occasional leap, as I did with QVC, I don't wing it. I am not that sort of person. I know some people who are very good at that and I watch them in awe, striding off to be brilliant without much prep or planning. It's enough to give me nightmares.

Occasionally, I have an anxiety dream where I find myself back at school and about to sit a chemistry exam. This is ludicrous because I never did the subject in real life, but as I sit down for the test, I realise everyone else around me has revised. They know what they are doing and I clearly don't.

Thankfully, I wake up before I am faced with a page of impossible equations, so I never have to put myself through the exam, but it is a regular reminder to focus. I always do my homework now, which is ironic considering my school days when I did the bare minimum for most of the time. Now I make notes before shows, underline sections with my highlighter pen and read something several times over. I will even condense information on to little cards in case I need to refer to them. I never do, but just knowing I have this as a back-up makes me feel safe.

Sometimes, I wonder if I *could* wing it. It might be fun in a risky sort of way, like riding a huge rollercoaster or leaving the house without my phone, which shows what sort of daredevil I am (not)! I wish I could have the confidence to do it and I am envious of those who do. I am not saying they don't put in the work, I just think they have a different attitude. More easy-breezy, seat-of-the-pants rather than prepared and over-organised. Some people thrive on taking a deadline up to the wire. I am not one of them. I don't like stress. I hate the feeling that I may get caught out.

My theory, particularly where my job is concerned, is that if something fails it won't be because I didn't put the work in. It's this sort of commitment that gives me confidence in whatever I am doing, whether it is creating my clothing range at QVC or presenting on live television.

I work with a fantastic team at QVC, and I don't want to let them down by being under-prepared. I owe it to them to be in the design meeting, test the samples and ask all the questions so by the time I get on air, I can talk knowledgeably about each garment and represent the work they have put in. The viewer sees me, but they do not see the team behind me making it all happen. That is my duty to the team, to my customers and to myself.

As for *Loose Women*, I always read the researchers' brief about the guests. Not only have they spent a lot of time putting it together, but they have also done it to help me and support the show. I can't watch and read everything so having information about our guests really helps. If I don't read it, then more fool me.

I have been a TV presenter for a long time and I know if push comes to shove and I am given a last-minute guest and no information, I could wing it. I have interviewed enough people over the years to be able to deal with this, but it isn't my chosen way of working. The fact is, I may be able to fudge it, but I don't want to.

But the older I get, the more I wonder. When I'm on a plane, I think I am the only person who is scared. I look at the other people – reading their books, watching a film – and nobody looks worried apart from me. But maybe lots of them are and they are just attempting to distract themselves. Maybe everyone is winging it a bit, and maybe I need to try. I take great inspiration from the people around me.

Iconic women in TV, like Gloria Hunniford and Janet Street-Porter, have been trailblazers and I have always benefited from seeing the generations ahead of me and learning from them. I look at those women and the careers they have had, and I listen to their stories, ask searching questions and soak up their advice like a sponge. I hope that younger generations remember this because, as we get older, we still have so much to share. Sometimes, I am aware of being dismissed and not being listened to, age making me invisible perhaps. I am sixty-six, I have a lot of experience, expertise and advice to offer, and I think those much younger than me would be wise to take note.

As a freelance presenter, I don't always have control over my career. What I can control is how hard I work and I thrive on the sense of purpose it gives me. That's why I always do my homework, read the papers to keep abreast of the news and watch the latest TV shows so I am match fit and ready to go. Being professional, respectful and well informed is what keeps me in the industry.

The confidence that comes from surviving everything life has thrown at us is invaluable. It's one of the better things about growing older. I know my capabilities, and I am sure of myself in many situations now. I don't fixate on what my peers, and those younger, are doing. I know where my career sits and although I would like nothing more, I probably won't be considered for a shiny-floor Saturday-night show. I am under no illusion about that, but to be honest that is quite a liberating place to be. No good comes from comparing ourselves to others, we need to forge ahead with our focus on what is right for us.

I am an enthusiastic cheerleader for younger presenters like my wonderful friend Rylan, who I hugely admire – I think he's a bit of a genius, actually. I wonder if he and his generation feel imposter syndrome like I did? I would love to hear their take on it.

Confidence is such a mercurial thing. One day you have it and the next it has disappeared in a puff of smoke. If this happens to me now, I try not to panic. I remind myself what I have achieved and that I am good enough. I want to share a couple of recent stories to illustrate this and how it all turned out OK in the end. And yes, while these are experiences that are unique to me and my job, I think they will resonate. It may be telly stuff for me, but it could be a work presentation, a wedding or a significant event for you.

So, having promised myself to start saying 'yes' to new things, I was invited on to Richard Osman's *House of Games*. This is a show that I love and take part in from the safety of my own sofa, often doing rather well, even if I do say so myself. If I was going to amble out of my comfort zone then this seemed like a good direction to head in and so I accepted, thought how lovely, popped it in the diary and promptly forgot about it.

Suddenly, it loomed, and with it came the terror of saying yes to something that I normally wouldn't have. What if I didn't get a single question right? What if everyone thought I was stupid? What on earth was I going to wear? Even trying to reassure myself with my dad's age-old 'what's the worst that can happen?' didn't calm my nerves.

My confidence and excitement about the opportunity began to ebb and in their place came all the fears and negativity, which then played out through my wardrobe planning for the filming week. I had five shows and needed to turn up with an outfit for each, plus a couple of spares in case I clashed with someone else. Easy, I do that all the time. Turned out it was more difficult than I expected.

I pulled out many possible outfits and tried them on. All I saw looking back at me in the mirror was a terrified, overweight and ancient woman; I had lost all reality in how I looked. Standing up, I didn't look too bad in some of the clothes I tried on, but the format of the show was to sit in a chair throughout the recordings and as soon as I did this, I thought I looked awful. This sent me into a spin about my middle-age spread, and I was one step away from throwing myself on to my bed to weep like a teenager.

I had ordered a khaki-coloured blazer, which I was pinning all my hopes on. I was waiting for it to arrive and when it didn't it felt like the company, the delivery driver and even the world was against me. I am well aware how ridiculous this all sounds, and that this was really about my fear of stepping into the unknown – I just hid behind the lack of outfit. I considered phoning the production team to say, 'Without the blazer, I can't go on!' I am not sure what I was thinking. Well, clearly I wasn't.

Every day I checked to see if the blazer had been delivered and sulked when it hadn't.

'You've got other blazers,' a friend pointed out.

'Yes, I know that,' I said grumpily, 'but I really need that green one.'

Extraordinary to look back on this and wonder how I had got myself in such a massive tizz that I couldn't get out of. I do a really good impression of myself stropping around about it, but at the time it was no laughing matter.

I called my stylist friend, Rachel, to ask for help and she offered to get a few items sent over to me, but what did I want? I didn't know, that was the problem, my mind was an utter blank. She suggested a couple of nice shirts and I said OK, but I wasn't convinced. The problem was that I was standing in front of a full rail of clothes and couldn't put together a single outfit, which was most unlike me. I was frozen in the face of what should have been a pretty simple task. Even when I put something on that looked vaguely OK, when I tried sitting down in it I instantly looked like a big sack of spuds.

It didn't help that I then watched a few episodes of the programme in an attempt to get in the mood and sat, silent and open-mouthed in horror, because I couldn't do any of the puzzles or word games. This hadn't happened before. I would have pulled out of the show if I could have done, and I was furious with myself for saying yes in the first place. Now I had to deal with the consequences.

Of course, the ten-act drama I made around choosing some clothes had very little to do with how I looked. I realised it was because I was so nervous about doing the show and I was convinced I was going to make a fool of myself. Wasn't I the one who messed around at school and left with only a handful of qualifications and a lack of general knowledge?! I had always turned down quiz shows so why was I suddenly booked to do one of the biggest on TV? Instead of understanding this and dealing with it, I let it become about a khaki blazer that hadn't arrived – when, deep down, I knew it was about my lack of confidence.

Even with the amount of telly experience I had and the extensive wardrobe of clothes I had literally designed myself, I felt completely out of my depth. It occurred to me that this show was a professional commitment I couldn't prep for, and I am a prepper. In fact, the only homework I could do was watch old shows back and this just made it worse because I didn't get the right answers and scared myself silly. I felt like the odds were stacked against me – but it was all OK in the end. Of course it was. Richard Osman is a superstar, I loved my time on the show, and I didn't let myself down. Am I glad I did it? Absolutely! And do you know what, when I got back the blazer had arrived. I tried it on and I hated it!

I get that the premise of the story isn't very relatable because it is about being on a TV show, but I think my behaviour is familiar and relevant in various situations. Perhaps you have accepted an invitation to a wedding or a party, knowing you have to go on your own, full of courage and conviction – until, that is, you get to the point where you are standing in front of your wardrobe. Women like me, whose lives have changed whether through menopause, a break-up or retirement maybe, are cautiously tiptoeing into a new stage. 'Who am I?' we ask and wait for a reply that will only come from inside ourselves. Not from a new blazer. Although sometimes that can help. We all have to get better at winging it.

Some people have an adventurous side and I don't. I am not afraid to admit this and there is no shame in it. I have never been on a rollercoaster, and you will absolutely never see me jump out of a plane or bungee off a bridge, attached to a bit of elastic rope. Why would I want to scare myself?! The only challenges I consider are connected with my career so it's hardly being outside of the box in a big way, but I am pushing myself.

My second example of this is when I hosted my very first 'Feeling Fabulous' event. When I was approached, the idea was presented as a fashion, beauty, fitness and well-being weekend, hosted by me at a great city venue. Something in that appealed and I thought, maybe I can do this – even though I had never done anything like it before, it tied together many elements of my career. I balked at the thought that it would be my name carrying the entire thing, but it didn't hurt to explore it.

Everything fell into place quite quickly, with QVC coming on board as a collaborator and sponsoring the catwalk section as well as several of my 'showbiz' friends agreeing to join me. This gave me an early confidence in the plan.

As the date got closer – tickets had been sold, stallholders booked and celebrities confirmed – I met the team, including the set designer, at the venue. We had settled on Old Billingsgate Market, overlooking the River Thames. I walked into this vast space, which to me felt the size of an aircraft hangar, and I felt sick. It was empty and I got the fear, but pretended to be as cool as a cucumber, as if I did this sort of thing all the time. In my head I was thinking, what the hell have I done? What have we done? It was just like planning the nursery and being in denial about a real baby arriving, I had not thought about actual people turning up. There we were talking about how the space would be filled, where to put the main stage, the beauty stage, the catwalk and the VIP area, and it was as much as I could do not to collapse under the weight of it all.

With a couple of weeks to go, I drove my management team mad with my worry over every single detail. I was in panic mode, while everyone involved told me it was going to be great, and then we all worked incredibly hard to make sure it was. There were several key issues that I did not want to compromise on, like good air conditioning and a coat and bag check-in because I knew what it was like to be a menopausal woman shuffling around in a crowd feeling a hot flush coming on. I had been to other events and felt overheated, too suffocated, and there was nowhere to leave my stuff, so I was lugging it around. That was not going to happen on my watch. The same with the number of loos. I hate having to queue, so we switched the ratio of toilets, creating more Ladies for the ladies. While I was keen to listen to the experts, I also knew what I wanted and led on certain points.

As the day drew closer and things became more stressful, I daydreamed about cancelling the whole thing. A couple of days before the event, one of the team asked me a perfectly simple question about choosing between two colours for the flowers, and I thought I was going to cry and then pass out with the stress of it all. If the event was a disaster, it would be me that everyone would blame, it was my name above the door and on the tickets, and I felt every minute of the pressure. I was full of foreboding.

The night before, I stayed with some of the QVC team in a hotel, where we had dinner together and then an early night. When I woke the following morning, a sense of calm came over me. There was nothing more to be done, we had achieved as much as we could and now it would be what it would be.

I was at the venue early and said hello and thank you to all the stallholders setting up before I dumped my stuff in a little room upstairs, where Liv and Maurice, my make-up and hair team, were setting up. Liv said there was a large queue forming outside and to come and take a look. Peeking out of a window I could see the tops of people's heads, standing in a long line, chatting to each other, some with takeaway coffees. The sun shone on the scene, and I was flooded with relief. Maybe it will be all right, I thought.

When I was hair and make-up ready, we walked down for the official opening, across a walkway above people who were already browsing around the stalls, and someone looked up and shouted, 'Hello Ruth!' and others waved. There was a sea of happy, smiling faces and from that moment on, I began to enjoy it.

As I dashed around between stages and events, women stopped me and we chatted. Time and time again I was told the same things: 'Thank you for doing this for us.' And 'There's nothing like this for us.' I realised the 'us' meant women over fifty. In organising the line-up, I had not wanted to be exclusive or intimidating, booking people who would take a relaxed, non-judgemental approach to fashion, cosmetics and fitness. Like my friend 'Fit with Frank', a personal trainer who runs online classes for people who are not confident about going to the gym, and he talked about how to incorporate exercise into our life as we age. And Donna May, a fantastic make-up artist who has created her own amazing brand and was sharing her easy-to-do make-up tips on the beauty stage. She is also a friend, and I loved being surrounded by familiar faces, but one was sadly missing.

My hairdresser was booked to do hair demos on the beauty stage, but unfortunately became unwell the night before. I was worried about him feeling so poorly but also now panicked about how to fill his slots . . . and then I thought of Liv and Maurice. So I texted them to explain what had happened and asked them if they would come on to the beauty stage with me, showing the audience how they did my hair and make-up for the various shows we work on together. I was pretty sure Liv would be happy to do it because she does a lot on Instagram, but Maurice is quite shy so I wasn't convinced he would say yes. True to form, Liv texted back within minutes to say she was happy to; Maurice took longer and agreed to do it as long as he could have a drink beforehand! Although he said he didn't want to speak, we kitted him out with a headset anyway and within a few minutes he was chatting away confidently, so much so we almost couldn't shut him up! They were both brilliant and ended up doing a demo on their own later in the day, getting audience members to come up on stage without me.

At the end of the second day, the final chat on the main stage was between Rylan and me, with Eamonn coming on with the drinks trolley as a surprise guest. We closed the event together, both of them urging me to take a walk down the runway to applause from the audience. It was crammed with women either side, some younger, but essentially my age group, all smiling and cheering. I thanked everyone for coming and I was so overwhelmed I burst into tears. I think the relief that the weekend was a success, coupled with the feeling in the room, surrounded by all these women, was uplifting and humbling. It took my breath away.

Afterwards, we had the most amazing feedback from our visitors, who loved everything from the beauty demos to the stalls to the speakers. My friend the perfumier Jo Malone was a big hit, as was my dancing partner Anton Du Beke, entrepreneur and crafting goddess Sara Davies, fashion journalist and editor Jo Elvin and telly pals Rylan, Vanessa Feltz and Jenni Falconer. I was particularly grateful to my dear friend and TV presenter Lucy Alexander for hosting the beauty stage and the fantastic Angellica Bell, who ran the main stage. QVC's fashion shows were a triumph, not just my brand but a great cross-section of collections hosted by Jackie and another wonderful colleague of ours, Melissa. The stallholders included brands like Jo Loves, Elemis, Donna May and IT Cosmetics, who were doing very popular ten-minute makeovers. Even my eighty-year-old Auntie Rosa came with a couple of her friends and said they had a whale of a time.

Indeed, it was the women who came that made the event. We may have set up the structure for them and paid attention to important details, but they brought the atmosphere and the energy. It felt like the beginning of something, the building of a community, and there is a desire and a plan to do it again so I hope, if we do, that I may see you there.

I was so glad I had been part of it and that I hadn't listened to the pessimistic voice in my head that told me to run in the opposite direction. My confidence was truly tested, but we had created an event that I would have wanted to be at as a visitor. And while I was incredibly proud of the team who worked tirelessly to make it a success, I was also proud of myself. It rested on my name, and I didn't let myself or anybody else down. The worst did not happen. Sometimes the best does.

16

On Being Fabulous

Well, here we are, the final chapter of this book, looking ahead to the next chapter of my life. Something tells me it's going to be good. I have a feeling it may be for you too. I am sixty-six years old and still I don't always have the answer, but that doesn't matter anymore.

When my marriage broke up, I kept wondering out loud, 'What is to become of me?' as if I was some Victorian lady with no prospects. I worried how I would survive. Well, Gloria Gaynor came up with the response to that one a long time ago and I didn't crumble and I didn't lay down and die. Instead, I gradually got myself back on track . . . I survived.

I still laugh when I think about that question, because what I was really saying was what was to become of me WITHOUT A HUSBAND. That seems faintly ridiculous now. I am not that person who has to be part of a couple. I have always made my own decisions and looked after myself so why would a divorce make any difference? When people refer to me as a strong, independent woman now my marriage is over, it makes it sound like I wasn't that before – but I always was, with or without a man.

Now I ask myself the same question in a completely different way. Now I am full of positive anticipation about 'what will become of me' because there is a whole world out there for me to explore.

Counselling has really helped me, and while I could consider mindfulness, meditation and journalling, which I know help so many people, it's not a natural place for me to be. My way of coping is to keep calm and carry on. Never say never, but I don't want to spend a lot of time visualising what I want for my future, I just want to live it. I have swung from fear of the unknown to trying to embrace it. I am getting there.

I am always busy doing something. If I'm not at ITV or QVC then I might be in my office working on my fashion collection, at a photoshoot, answering emails, discussing projects with my agent or writing notes for the next live show (or book!). I work hard but then so do a lot of people and I have no complaints because I am doing what I love. Work has been my saviour and my sanctuary over the years, and I hope it will continue long into my future.

By the weekend, I am tired, so they are precious, and I try not to do anything work-related. I always see Mum, she loves coming around to see Maggie and we visit her at the care home too. I never get bored at home and I cherish an evening on my own.

I love being organised, I think it is my superpower! There is such satisfaction when I know I have a free day to sort out a room, unpack boxes of clothes from QVC or prep for the week ahead. Having time like this always makes me feel back in control. Sometimes I don't realise how stressed I am about the chaos until I have a couple of clear days and can get everything sorted.

Occasionally when I have finished a job, like reorganising my airing cupboard perhaps, I find myself going back to have a look. That's how happy it makes me! I have even been known to add things to my running to-do list that I've already done, just so I can have the pleasure of ticking them off. I imagine some of you are telling me to 'get a life' right now (looking at you, Coleen!), but this is the life I am happy in. Not sexy, but there we are. At least I know where all my sheets are and that they are clean and neatly folded.

I live by my online diary, which my team has access to. You will know by now that I am not an out-of-control kind of girl. I feel lost without routine. I am not disorganised and if I ever find myself becoming so, then I would have to change something in my life immediately because I know how much I hate the feeling – I imagine it feels like being on a runaway horse. I always pack my bag the night before ready for whatever I am doing the next day, and make sure I have everything I need, then I am off-duty for the evening. I even put a teabag in my mug and make sure the kettle is full, ready to make my first cuppa in the morning. Every second counts!

If I have a week off, I tend to go away, otherwise I would be elbows deep in chores at home because I can't help myself. It's much harder to switch off there, but when I can escape I find it easy to relax, and lazy holidays – where all I have to do is lie by the pool, read, drink cocktails, eat and sleep – are my favourite. That's why I don't always go somewhere with amazing history and ancient monuments because then I feel I should be sightseeing. I save those cultural experiences for weekend city breaks and then I have my sunbathing holidays for chilling out and spending time with Jack or my girls.

I can't imagine retiring for a long time, that's not something I have any desire to do, and I know I am not alone in this, particularly when many of us still have bills to pay. If the television industry gave me up tomorrow, I would feel terribly sad about it and it would knock the wind out of my sails, but I have navigated worse. I think I am good at my job, and I have a natural curiosity about people so it's a privilege to do what I do, but if my live telly days were over, I would hope to use those skills in whatever I did next. I would still want to work because it's an environment I thrive in. As well as being quite a creative person, I could see myself being useful in a garden centre because I'm always happy when I am in one and I enjoy pottering around my own garden. I think it's in my DNA as the women in my family have been the same.

Where do I see myself in five years from now? I haven't a clue. As organised as I am in my day-to-day, I am not someone who maps out the rest of their life. I don't think in terms of what I will do for the year ahead. It's enough for me to focus on the next month, indeed even the next week. I hope I will still be working doing what I love and that I will be fit and healthy. More than that, I cannot say. I often think if you plan too much, you can disappoint yourself. It's good to have goals but not to be so restricted by them that you feel bad if you don't achieve everything.

Quite early on, my counsellor said, 'Ruth, your marriage is over, and you won't be able to see the light and move forward until you accept that.' And she was right, but I had to go through the grieving process first. Like they always say, after the darkness comes the dawn. Heartbreak is heartbreak but it's not going to kill you.

I have impressed myself. I know I shouldn't say this, but I look at myself now and what I have been through, and I say, 'Do you know what, Ruth, bloody well done!' I didn't lose myself. I sat in the initial shock followed by the upset and then the uncomfortable and I kept going. Day after day. I hung on to the negative things for a while but now I try to look only for the positives.

Several times recently I have been asked if I'm back on the dating scene and it bemuses me, because why would I want to jump into a new relationship when I'm still dealing with the emotional fallout of the old one? Someone asked if I was looking for Mr Right and I thought, isn't that a rather old-fashioned concept? Plus, I thought I had found my soulmate, my Mr Right, and look what happened there. While I don't think that a woman needs a man to be happy, it's important to say that I have not been put off relationships or even marriage, but neither am I out there looking for a new partner.

I didn't expect to be single at this stage of my life, but here I am. I didn't expect not to have my sister, either, or for my mum to have Alzheimer's. There is no changing it and I'm not making any big, bold moves or significant plans, I am just ready for whatever is next.

Life doesn't finish in middle age. It can begin. Whether you are forty or sixty, in a relationship or not, working hard or heading to retirement, settling in at home or ready to travel, every single day is precious. Sometimes we just need a little nudge or a few wise words to keep us steady.

These are things I say to myself that may help you . . .

- Don't panic – simple but effective. I never look like I am panicking but I can feel it in my gut and I have to remind myself it's wasting energy.
- No sudden moves – as an organiser, it is so tempting to Make Plans and Keep Busy. In my experience, a knee-jerk reaction will give you the wrong result. I have learned to sit on my hands during those times. Don't cut your hair, change career or sell your house until you're sure you are making those decisions for the right reasons.
- Hold steady – similar to the above, but directed more at the emotion of a situation rather than the practical. It's a good thing to say to your nervous system.
- Don't look back – nothing is gained from going over the past in forensic detail, raging against what could have been and where things went wrong. The same goes for being stuck in a time when we were happiest. We need to forge ahead to find the next joy – like being in the sea and treading water in a cold spot, let's swim on to find the warmth.
- Carry on with what you are doing – let's not spend our lives looking left or right at what others are up to. They are on their own quest; you are on yours. Don't be distracted by people you perceive are more successful and therefore happier, because that often isn't the case. Let's all remember what Anton told me and be ourselves.
- You don't have to do anything crazy – when big things happen in our lives, we can feel drawn to showing we are still alive or taking on challenges we would never have

On Being Fabulous

considered. So, no, you don't have to skydive, move to another country or take up marathon running.
- This is your life – it's not your children's, or your partner's or your parents'. It's yours. It may seem ridiculous to remind you of this, but I think we all forget it at times.
- Stay in the moment and see where it takes you – I tell myself this a lot because I find it the hardest thing to do, but I am getting much better at it.

Being fabulous encapsulates so many things for me. As we have already discussed, it's not just about how we look, it's a feeling. We each need to find our own fabulous and think about what it means to us. It can be the smallest thing, like your first coffee in the morning, not just the big showy stuff. Sometimes it may be so tiny you could miss it, so we all need to tune into ourselves and find out where that feeling comes from. These are some of mine . . .

- Taking Maggie out for a walk, a daily joy. I always take my phone, just in case, but I try to leave it in my pocket so I am not tempted to scroll. I want to immerse myself in the season, breathe deeply, look at the trees and enjoy Maggie's delight at being outside. This is my fabulous.
- Being with my friends, at home or on holiday, drinking gin and laughing until we cry. This is my fabulous.
- Sitting on my sofa in my slobs with the fire on and the theme tune for *Coronation Street* starting up. This is my fabulous.
- Getting dressed up and going out with friends for a long

lunch that turns into early-evening cocktails. This is my fabulous.
- Being on my own in the kitchen, batch cooking or prepping ready to feed people. This is my fabulous.

And just to expand on this (and take a short detour from the list) because food has been a small, insistent thread throughout this book, I find thinking about it incredibly therapeutic, as is making it, whether it's for a group or just for me. In a parallel life I live in a big farmhouse with a huge kitchen, and I cook all the time. In my actual life, I always enjoy making my packed lunches to take into work or brewing my ginger tea recipe if I am a bit run down. It feeds my soul. If we eat to live or live to eat, I fall into the latter category. One of my greatest joys is to have my favourite music turned up loud and be slicing, blending and frying. It never feels like a chore.

Even on my down days, I can lose myself in making soup. In that moment, as I am chopping and stirring, I push the sadness to one side and focus on making delicious food. Making it is just as nourishing for my soul as eating it is for my body, as is the warm hug of a smell that fills the kitchen.

I don't entertain and throw dinner parties in a formal sense anymore. I don't think I did many, although there has been the odd occasion over the years when I have pulled out all the stops. You know, the linen tablecloth, polished-until-shining cutlery, matching glassware and flickering candles set out ready for a four-course feast that I would have spent the day slaving over.

This reminds me of the time I made champagne sorbet

and was serving it in frosted glasses, with a decoration of candied (sugary) grapes, bringing it out just after the main course. They looked pretty impressive as I moved around the table handing them out. I went to put one in front of a woman, the wife of someone I didn't know very well, who, without even looking at it, said dismissively, 'Not for me, thanks.' Not for me? NOT FOR ME?! Had she seen it? Did she realise how long it had taken me? I was tempted to dump it on her haughty head.

Now I realise that nobody really cares. It isn't about impressing people, I just want my friends to have a good time. The food is secondary to that. As long as what we eat is delicious, I don't need to spend hours in the kitchen. Sometimes the best supper to share is a big lasagne, or a couple of roast chickens served with a big salad and a pile of garlic bread. Nobody wants me stuck in the kitchen all evening, frosting glasses for a sorbet! Although I still make an effort with the table because that elevates a kitchen supper into more of an occasion, particularly if it is for someone's birthday. Now if that isn't a vital lesson learned, I don't know what is. No more champagne sorbets. Or maybe no more people around my table who I don't know!

And just to return to my list for my two most important points . . .

- o Seeing Mum's face light up when Maggie and I come to visit. This is my fabulous.
- o Jack coming home for the weekend and cooking breakfast for him while he sits at the breakfast bar, chatting to me. This is my fabulous.

So, there is my list of some of the things I do that make me feel fabulous. They may not be yours, so find out what they are. What is it that makes you happy and content? Figure this out and do as much of it as you can. You could even note them down as I have done here. You know how much I love a list! It doesn't hurt to remind ourselves of the good stuff as much as we remind ourselves about the chores we have to do.

Thank you for being with me as I recount some of the worst, most painful times of my life as well as spread the importance of love, friendship, family, work and purpose, and not forgetting the glorious frippery of fashion, food and fun times. I have lived it all and while there are a few experiences I never want to repeat, for the most part it's been a happy life, and I am looking forward to what might be next.

So, go and live the life you want. Be brilliant, be fabulous and be free to be you. As for the life I want? It's on the horizon and I am excited with a small 'e'.

The other morning, I was standing in my kitchen looking out of the window. It was a beautiful day, the sun was streaming in, filling the room with its positive warmth. I had music on in the background and the coffee machine was gurgling away. Maggie was snoozing in her bed and the day stretched out luxuriously in front of me with no plans. I realised that this feeling I had was contentment, I was happy. This hadn't been a conscious thought; it came over me in a quiet moment of reflection and peace. It has been hard won, and yet here I am. And I can't wait to see what will become of me.

Acknowledgements

I'd like to thank everyone at Hodder & Stoughton, including Kate Miles, Becca Mundy, Inayah Sheikh Thomas and Jazmin Demjan for their unerring support and encouragement knowing how nervous I was about writing this book. Special thanks to my editor Susannah Otter, who I loved from the moment I met her and who convinced me people would want to read my story!

To writer, and now friend, Lucy Brazier who was with me on this literary path. We laughed, we cried, we mused and we drank coffee together – and without her this book would have been much harder to write.

To my management at YMU including Briony, Sarah, Jack and Bridie and Lou from Plank PR . . . thank you for always believing in me and for continuing to bang on about me doing a book until I did something about it! I cursed you all many times during this process, but I will be eternally grateful.

To my wonderful friends for their unconditional love and support. There are so many times in my life I wouldn't have survived without you. You know who you are . . . I love you all. Sorry I wasn't around much to drink wine while writing this book . . . we will be back to business now!

Feeling Fabulous

Finally, to my darling son Jack. Thank you for being the best son a mother could have and for allowing me to write about you without complaining it was 'cringe'! You'll find out a bit more about your Mum if you bother to read it! I love you more than you'll ever know.

RAISING READERS
Books Build Bright Futures

Dear Reader,

We'd love your attention for one more page to tell you about the crisis in children's reading, and what we can all do.

Studies have shown that reading for fun is the **single biggest predictor of a child's future life chances** – more than family circumstance, parents' educational background or income. It improves academic results, mental health, wealth, communication skills, ambition and happiness.[1]

The number of children reading for fun is in rapid decline. Young people have a lot of competition for their time. In 2024, 1 in 10 children and young people in the UK aged 5 to 18 did not own a single book at home.[2]

Hachette works extensively with schools, libraries and literacy charities, but here are some ways we can all raise more readers:

- Reading to children for just 10 minutes a day makes a difference
- Don't give up if children aren't regular readers – there will be books for them!
- Visit bookshops and libraries to get recommendations
- Encourage them to listen to audiobooks
- Support school libraries
- Give books as gifts

There's a lot more information about how to encourage children to read on our website: **www.RaisingReaders.co.uk**

Thank you for reading.

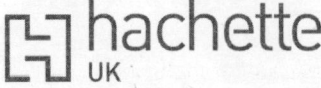

---

[1] OECD, '21st-Century Readers: Developing Literacy Skills in a Digital World', 2021, https://www.oecd.org/en/publications/21st-century-readers_a83d84cb-en.html

[2] National Literacy Trust, 'Book Ownership in 2024', November 2024, https://literacytrust.org.uk/research-services/research-reports/book-ownership-in-2024